How Weight Loss Surgery Really Works

AND HOW TO MAKE IT WORK FOR YOU

MATTHEW WEINER, MD

To my parents who've always been there for us.

First Edition: August 2019
Printed in the United States of America
ISBN: 9781688128804

This book is not intended to replace advice from a physician. If you have any medical conditions or symptoms that are concerning, a physician should be consulted, rather than relying on the information found within this book. This book represents the current state of medical knowledge as of August 2019. As more research becomes available, some of the information in this book may become invalid. You should seek the most up to date information from a physician or other health care professional.

Table of Contents

ACKNOWLEDGEMENTS

This book would not have been possible without the trust of my patients over the last decade. By sharing your stories with me and showing the courage that going through weight loss surgery requires, you've offered me an opportunity to learn more about obesity and weight loss surgery than I ever could from any textbook, mentor or scientific paper. I'd also like to thank Ruby Weiner, age 12 who helped with many of the illustrations found in this book.

CHAPTER ONE
INTRODUCTION

I've been a bariatric surgeon for twelve years and have performed over 2,000 weight loss surgeries. Even more importantly, I estimate that I've had around 4,000 thirty-minute conversations with patients about what caused their weight gain, the things they've done to try to lose weight, and what their hopes and fears are surrounding their decision to undergo weight loss surgery.

Obesity does not discriminate by age, gender, socioeconomic class or personality type. These conversations have been matter-of-fact discussions of the latest research with a 53-year-old married engineer and his wife and tearful and intensely personal discussions with a 27-year-old single woman about all the ways her obesity has negatively influenced her life. Overcoming obesity is not easy and requires a complete and thorough change in your understanding of not just weight loss surgery, but also, the underlying causes of weight gain and weight loss. It requires you to think about obesity in a completely new way and expunge the "calorie in/calorie out" model from your brain.

Several million people in the United States have undergone weight loss surgery and their successes have transformed our understanding of weight gain and weight loss. Rather than looking at obesity as a personal failure caused by a lack of willpower, we are starting to understand that obesity is a disease of fat storage that shares many characteristics with other chronic diseases like diabetes, high blood pressure, and heart disease.

In my opinion, the first step that prospective weight loss surgery patients should take is to completely discard the notion that their weight gain is primarily driven by a lack of willpower. Most of my patients are successful in other aspects of their life. They're a faithful spouse, dedicated employee, and committed parent who is able to express discipline in every facet of their life- except when it comes to losing weight. Most of my patients can't grasp the dichotomy between their failures on the bathroom scale and their success on all other fronts until they begin to look at obesity for what it really is. ***Obesity is a disease that causes a breakdown in the regulation of your fat stores and is the result of a person's genetics and life experiences.*** Willpower plays a very small and relatively insignificant role in this process. Viewing your past struggles with your weight through this lens is the only way to come to terms with a lifetime of weight loss failure.

I started my career in Bariatric Surgery with the same misconceived notions that pervade our popular culture; obesity is a disease of eating too much and exercising too little. I initially prescribed low calorie processed foods and protein shakes for my patients and cheered them on with motivational speeches so that they would finally decide to change their lives. However, in many of these conversations, patients shared details of their daily habits that directly conflicted with the way I was looking at weight gain. Many of my patients were eating fewer calories than I did and exercising more frequently yet weighed 100 lbs. more. Around the same time I began to notice this contradiction, a growing number of research papers were published that directly challenged our notion of calorie balance as the primary determinant of obesity.[1,2,3]

The "new" science of weight gain has changed my belief that obesity is a lifestyle choice and is the direct result of the overconsumption of calories. Instead, weight gain and obesity are the result of a derangement of physiology, rather than of willpower. These physiologic changes parallel those that are seen in high blood pressure, diabetes, high cholesterol, and most other chronic diseases. By looking at obesity as an alteration in your brain, gut, and fat store physiology, rather than a behavioral disease, many of our commonly held conceptions about your diet after weight loss surgery, eating behaviors, and weight regain no longer make much sense. I was seeing the truth in the "new" science at work in my practice and the more I learned, the more answers I was able to offer my patients.

As I read the research studies that demonstrated the impact of nutrition, genetics, and bariatric surgery on appetite, body weight, and fat storage, I slowly revamped my pre-operative educational program to include a concept that I referred to as your "metabolic thermostat" which will be described in detail in later chapters. My patients immediately embraced the idea of a mechanism that regulated their body weight and worked in opposition to their attempts at weight loss. When I took a detailed history, I found that we were nearly always able to identify specific life events that had raised the set point on their metabolic thermostat resulting in 10, 15, or even more pounds added to their waistline that were entirely resistant to their dieting efforts.

Once I stopped looking at the world through a calorie and willpower lens and started to use the metabolic thermostat to guide my treatment decisions and advice, a few pretty amazing things happened. First, I was able to unburden patients from the guilt and shame that their losing battle against the scale had left behind. Second, my relationship with my patients strengthened. When weight gain is viewed as an elevation of your metabolic thermostat's set point, rather than the result of a lack of self-control, the doctor becomes the partner- not the accuser. Third, I questioned the wisdom of many of the rules that are presented to bariatric surgery patients as gospel. The idea of eating protein first and living on mega-doses of supplemental shakes made far less sense than focusing on fruits, vegetables, nuts, seeds, and beans as the backbone of their postoperative diet.

In short, my new and improved view of weight loss and bariatric surgery changed everything that I did for my patients outside of the operating room. The reports I was getting from patients about their appetite, energy level, and cravings for different foods now made sense and fit tightly with my new appreciation for the hormonal changes brought about by these surgeries.

Weight loss surgery is a true 21st century modern miracle that is slowly changing our view of weight gain and obesity. I continue to be amazed by the transformations I see in my office every day as a I watch my patients shed hundreds of pounds, come off dozens of medications, start exercising regularly and eat a diet consisting primarily of fruits, vegetables, nuts, seeds, beans, and lean animal protein. There is much myth and lore that surrounds these surgeries and much of it continues to pervade the online communities, popular press, and even the recommendations of many bariatric surgery programs. My approach to weight loss surgery attempts to dispel these inaccuracies and offers patients a strategy for success after surgery that is guided by research, common sense, and my clinical experiences. Many of the recommendations may be counterintuitive at a superficial level and only make sense as we delve deeper into the complex disease of obesity. In the end, I find that the best patients are the ones who put in the time to educate themselves about weight loss surgery. I hope this book offers a guiding philosophy that serves as the scaffold on which you build your understanding of weight loss, weight gain and Bariatric Surgery.

CHAPTER TWO
YOUR METABOLIC THERMOSTAT

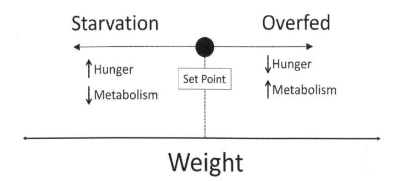

Figure 1 - Your Metabolic Thermostat

In my first book, *A Pound of Cure*, I introduced the idea of a metabolic thermostat that controls your body weight. Just like the thermostat in your house that controls the temperature of the room by delivering either cold or warm air in response to the ambient temperature, your metabolic thermostat adjusts your hunger and metabolic rate in response to your body weight. This concept views your excess body fat as a tightly controlled physiologic parameter, rather than a simple receptacle for extra calories. Your metabolic thermostat regulates your hunger, metabolic rate, food choices, and willingness to exercise through a complicated interplay between your brain, gut, fat stores, circulating hormones, and nervous system.

Before going into the details of how your body works to regulate your fat stores, let's discuss the way your body works to control other vital physiological parameters like your heart rate, blood pressure, or blood glucose level. There is a tight network of sensors throughout your body that work to detect changes in a vital parameter (like your heart rate, blood pressure or blood glucose level) and trigger feedback responses to restore the parameter back to the normal level and maintain a steady state. The medical term for this concept is *homeostasis* which loosely translates to "stay the same."

A classic example of homeostasis at work is your blood pressure, immediately after you stand up. The moment you stand, your blood will pool in your legs and cause a drop in your blood pressure. This will be detected by the millions of sensors that exist in your blood vessels and will trigger an immediate response to increase your heart rate, narrow your blood vessels, and make your heart beat stronger, all to counteract this blood pressure drop[4,5]. The result will be your blood pressure returning to normal within a fraction of a second after you stand up. As the blood that has pooled in your legs begins to circulate again, your blood pressure will return to normal, your heart rate will slow down, the blood vessels will squeeze less, and your heart will go back to its normal contractile strength[6]. This feedback loop and hundreds of others is vital to our body's inner workings.

When we look at our body's regulation of hunger and metabolism, we find a similar system that works to preserve our precious fat stores through periods of famine or starvation[7,8]. Fortunately, starvation is not a problem we face today in the Western world, but our physiology has not yet gotten this message. In the modern world, our body's response to starvation is now triggered predominantly by our attempts at weight loss, rather than its intended function, to prevent us from dying of malnutrition[9].

All of us have a particular body weight that we tend to center around from week to week or even month to month. One week you may eat healthier, exercise more, and drop a few pounds. The following week, you lose focus and your weight drifts back up, but it will usually center around a predetermined, specific weight. This is because your metabolic thermostat has a set point that regulates your fat stores to keep them relatively stable over time. Your body weight, just like your blood pressure is maintained via feedback loops through the process of homeostasis[7].

When the change in your dieting and exercise habits is more significant, your metabolic thermostat shifts into overdrive. During periods of starvation (dieting), you will lose a few pounds which causes your body weight to drop below the set point. This drop will trigger feedback loops within your metabolic thermostat to work to restore the lost weight by increasing your brain's focus on food (hunger) and by slowing your metabolism down to reduce your body's need for calories[9].

If you've ever thought that your body was set on preventing you from losing weight - you were right. It's important to remember that our body's physiology has evolved over hundreds of thousands of years. A caveman who did not experience much hunger had little desire to brave the snow and rain to go out to hunt and forage for food. This did not bode well for his survival. Furthermore, those individuals that could not down-regulate their metabolic rate in response to periods of starvation did not stand a chance of making it through the long, cold winter without burning up their excess fat stores. A caveman's survival was directly linked to his ability to survive on a few hundred calories a day during those periods of famine that inevitably occurred each year. These same forces that ensured our ancestors' survival ten thousand years ago are now working directly against us as we try to lose weight by restricting our calorie intake.

It is only over the last fifty years that diabetes and obesity has become a bigger risk than starvation. Physiologic and genetic changes take many, many generations to change, so your metabolic thermostat continues to function as it has for the last ten thousand years and works to minimize your risk of dying of malnutrition even though this is no longer a legitimate concern.

We've all been told that weight loss is driven by willpower and the discipline to resist our hunger drive, but this is difficult if not impossible for most of us. Resisting a physiologic drive is possible for short periods of time but, uniformly, will fail in the long run. Let's use the same willpower argument that is used to explain why dieters fail and apply it to a similar exercise in resisting your physiologic drive – holding your breath. All of us can hold our breath for 10 seconds and resist our brain's drive to breathe. After 20 seconds, many of us will start to experience significant air hunger and be unable to focus on anything except getting your next breath. At 30 seconds, one minute, or even two minutes for the most determined, we will eventually succumb to our physiological drive for oxygen and will give up and take a breath.

Resisting your hunger over time is a similar exercise in futility. Many of us can ignore our hunger for several weeks, and the more disciplined for several months. But inevitably, as our body weight drops and our metabolic thermostat releases stronger and stronger hunger signals, our constant exposure to food will win out and we will stray from our 1200 calorie a day diet. As we will discuss later, this does not mean that you cannot lose weight by modifying your food intake, it just means that simply reducing your calorie intake is not the way to do it in the long run.

Like all the other systems in our body, there is never just one way that our physiology works to preserve our fat stores. In addition to modifying your hunger in response to periods of decreased calorie intake, your body will also adjust the rate that it burns calories. When you reduce your calorie intake, your metabolic thermostat works to decrease the rate that you burn calories[10]. This explains why you lose 4-5 pounds the first week (on a 1200 calorie a day diet), 1-2 pounds the next few weeks, and eventually "plateau" and stop losing weight without changing your diet at all. Eventually, your metabolic thermostat changes your metabolic rate to ensure that you are only burning 1200 calories a day so that you don't lose any more of your precious fat stores. Your caveman survival techniques are triggered to preserve your fat stores and resist your attempts at weight loss. Even if you are motivated and go to the gym every day, get on the treadmill, set it to calorie mode and walk or run until the machine tells you that you've burned 300 calories, your metabolic thermostat will adjust to this increased calorie expenditure by down-regulating your metabolic rate even further that night as you sleep, directly sabotaging your weight loss efforts[11,12].

The increase in our hunger and slowing of our metabolic rate in response to starvation is something that all of us understand since we've experienced it first-hand. However, there is another side to our metabolic thermostat that works in exactly the opposite way. If we gain a few extra pounds, a healthy metabolic thermostat will work to normalize our body weight back to our set point[13]. We will decrease our hunger and find we have little interest in food[14]. Additionally, we will be triggered to move more, take the stairs, and walk further and faster in an effort to increase our metabolic rate. We see this each New Year after the winter holiday feasts result in a few (or more) pounds of weight gain. Come January 1st, most of us have a body weight a few pounds above our set point. Our metabolic thermostat responds by decreasing our hunger so that complying with that 800 calorie a day fad diet seems like a reasonable undertaking.

Our metabolism is also increased, so waking up early to go to the gym seems like a good idea. We're all convinced that this year is going to be the year we finally get rid of those extra pounds. That is until we lose a few pounds and drift below our set point. The hunger returns with a vengeance and our metabolism downshifts making us more likely to press the snooze button than wake up for that early morning workout.

The overfed functionality of our metabolic thermostat is as important as the starvation side for two reasons. First, bariatric surgery works by harnessing this side of the thermostat so that our physiology is working to drive weight loss - not prevent it. Second, it's a malfunction of this side of the thermostat that results in weight gain in the first place.

Whether we choose to lose weight by having weight loss surgery, changing our diet, exercising, or even taking medications, **we have to ensure that we are working to lower our metabolic thermostat's set point, rather than trying to fight against it.** If we can lower our set point below our current body weight, the overfed functionality will drive our physiology to decrease our hunger and increase our metabolism. This is the holy grail of weight loss. A lowered set point results in our body actually helping us to lose weight rather than fighting against us.

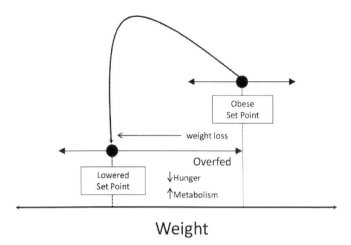

Weight

Figure 2- A lowered set point triggers the overfed side of your metabolic thermostat

One last important point about our metabolic thermostat concerns its "width." Most people are able to lose around 10% of their total body weight before the increase in hunger and decrease in their metabolic rate becomes insurmountable[15,16,17]. I've found this fact to be uncannily accurate. A 250-pound woman is usually able to lose 25 pounds before she loses focus and starts to regain weight. Most patients will point to external factors like stress in their job, travel or a "lack of willpower" when they discuss the reason why their diet and exercise habits changed; however, the dominant factor is their underlying physiologic drive to preserve their fat stores.

While the width of most people's metabolic thermostat is around 10%, there are a few exceptions. First, young people are often able to lose 20% or more of their body weight before they begin to hit the dreaded plateaus that ultimately sabotage even the most determined dieter[18]. Men seem to be more resistant to the impact of age on the width of their thermostat. Most women begin to lose their ability to lose more than 10% of their body weight in their 30's (often after pregnancy) while men are often able to extend this into their 40's.

There is also a subset of people (around 10% by my estimate) that preserve their ability to lose and maintain more than 25% of their body weight through calorie restriction[19]. This is likely the small group of people who do find success living by the "eat less, exercise more" approach to weight loss. There is little understanding of the physiologic factors that make these people resistant to the hunger and metabolism changes that occur as a result of starvation that plague the rest of us. For this unique group, obesity may in fact be a lifestyle choice. When they clean up their diet and exercise calorie restriction and portion control, they lose weight effortlessly, without plateaus. When they consume large amounts of calorie dense foods, they develop significant obesity. Unfortunately, our society sees the success and failure of these folks and extrapolates it to the rest of us. I am completely convinced that the majority of us are unable to lose and maintain more than 10% of our total body weight through traditional dieting methods. If you are among this majority, your focus cannot be on developing better methods of starving yourself. Instead you should focus on how to lower your body's set point.

Before we start to explore the ways that we can lower our metabolic thermostat's set point, we must first examine the reasons that our set point becomes elevated in the first place. Any attempts to lose weight must start by eliminating all factors that trigger set point elevation. Weight loss is hard enough without having to fight against medications, food addictions, or other factors that are raising our set point and triggering our body to increase its fat stores.

CHAPTER THREE
WHY YOU GAINED WEIGHT

It's extremely likely that, at some point in your life, you've been told that your weight gain is the result of your individual choices and inability to regulate your food intake and remain active. While this may be true in a few circumstances, it is a far more complex problem for most of the people that I see in my office. It turns out that our environment has a powerful influence on our daily decisions about food and exercise. Food marketers have known this for decades. They know that their product sells better if it is placed on shelves at eye level or on end caps, or in the most desirable of all locations, the checkout line. Our diet is strongly influenced by the way foods are organized in our local grocery store.

Our decisions about exercise and movement are also based strongly on our environment. If you don't have a car and your workplace is 2 miles away, you're much more likely to get your 10,000 steps in than if you own a car and commute 30 minutes each way to work. People who live in two-story houses climb a lot more stairs than those who live in ranch style homes.

Our environment also has very strong influences on other chronic conditions like high blood pressure[20], elevated cholesterol[21], diabetes[22], and heart disease[23]. Despite this, we do not place the same burden of responsibility on diabetics or those who have suffered a heart attack that we do on those who suffer from obesity. It would be completely unacceptable in our society to tell a patient admitted to the Emergency Room with a heart attack that it's their own fault that they're suffering because of their diet. In our society, heart disease triggers get well cards and thoughts and prayers, while obesity brings out derisive looks and careless comments intended to shame. However, if we carefully consider the real causes of obesity, we find that they are incredibly similar to those that cause heart disease.

When I meet with new patients, I spend quite a bit of time diving into the reasons behind their weight gain. What does your food and exercise environment look like? When did your weight gain start? Are there others in your family who struggle with their weight? What medications did you take in the past? Have you ever suffered an injury that resulted in a prolonged period of inactivity? These questions are critical to understanding why each patient has gained weight and guides what we do in the future to minimize factors that may interfere with future weight loss efforts.

While the choices that you make about what you eat and whether or not you exercise are very important, they are not the only factors that determine whether or not you gain weight. Let's start by reviewing the most common causes of weight gain that I see in my practice.

Medications

Approximately one-third of the patients that I see in my office are taking or have taken medications that list weight gain as a side effect. Many have been told that the weight gaining effects of the medication can be prevented by strict adherence to a diet. This recommendation flies directly in the face of research that demonstrates that weight gain induced by medications is difficult to prevent[24]. Prescribing physicians often point to their experience with a few patients who did not gain weight on these medications as an example of how strict discipline can counteract this side effect. These individual examples are not useful counterpoints since the weight gaining side effects are not experienced by 100% of the patients. Just because one patient did not gain weight from taking a certain medication does not mean that you won't either. My experience is that patients who are not significantly overweight are more resistant to weight gain from medications than those who are fifty or more pounds overweight.

Now that we have a solid understanding of our metabolic thermostat, the idea that a medication can cause weight gain is easier to understand. If you are taking a medication every day that alters any part of the relationship between your brain, gut, fat stores, and hunger and metabolism regulating hormones, it could slowly raise your set point and trigger your metabolism to slow down and increase your fat stores. It will also likely increase your appetite. This can be resisted - at least at first. However, the impact on your metabolic rate is much less modifiable. Even if you head to the gym every day in an attempt to prevent the weight gain from the medication, the other factors that work to slow down your metabolic rate will be unaffected[25]. Your weight loss efforts will be futile. Your decreased calorie consumption will trigger even greater hunger and your efforts in the gym will be thwarted every evening as you burn fewer calories in your sleep. **Most people focus their weight loss efforts by taking actions to drive weight loss, however, your success is equally dependent on your ability to eliminate lifestyle factors (like unnecessary medications) that cause set point elevation.**

If a medication triggers set point elevation, you will quickly find yourself in the equivalent position of someone who has just completed a month-long starvation diet. Your body weight will be below your set point and your physiology will work to drive your body weight upward until it gets back to your set point. Most of us have experienced the rapid weight regain that occurs when we return to our regular eating pattern after an extremely restrictive diet. This same effect is triggered when a medication causes set point elevation, but instead of returning to our normal weight, we gain weight to match our new elevated set point.

Most medications do not trigger set point elevation and even if you are taking a medication that does, it is important that you discuss this with your prescribing physician before stopping the medication. Many of these medications cannot be stopped immediately and must be tapered slowly to prevent dangerous side effects. Let's review a few of the most common weight gaining medications out there.

Depo-Provera®: This medication is an injection that serves as a long-acting form of birth control. It is one of the most potent weight gaining medications on this list and I've met many patients who have gained fifty or more pounds from it. In my opinion, any patient who is at all concerned about her weight should avoid the use of this form of birth control. Pregnancy typically results in set point elevation in order to increase a woman's fat stores to ensure that she is able to provide adequate nutrition to a developing fetus. Depo-Provera® stimulates a similar hormonal state to pregnancy and triggers the same pattern of weight gain[26]. It's important to note that most daily birth control pills do not trigger the same hormonal changes and do not need to be avoided. If you are struggling with your weight and are deciding on a method for birth control, please make sure that you discuss this with your doctor to ensure that your weight loss efforts are not inhibited by your choice of birth control.

Corticosteroids: Prednisone is the most common form of corticosteroid, but there are several others that induce the same effects. Steroids are incredibly useful and often lifesaving medications that are used to treat asthma, inflammatory bowel disease, and many autoimmune conditions like Lupus and Rheumatoid Arthritis. While they are very effective, they typically cause a significant disruption in your body fat storage. They can trigger 20-30 pounds of weight gain per year and trigger an increase in your appetite that is almost impossible to control[27]. They are often prescribed in short bursts which typically do not cause significant weight gain until patients are using them 3-4 times per year. There are more and more medications available to treat the same conditions that don't cause weight gain, so be sure to discuss all your options with your physician before starting a steroid regimen.

Mood Stabilizing Medications for Bipolar Disorder: Obesity is more prevalent in patients with Bipolar disorder[28] and we have observed that patients who suffer from Bipolar disorder lose less weight after bariatric surgery[29]. While the science is incomplete on this point, most physicians suspect that the medications used to treat these conditions are a major factor in its correlation with obesity. Again, it is critical to work with your prescribing physician on the optimal regimen to control your mood disorder and limit weight gain.

The weight gaining effects are not experienced by all patients, so you may be able to tolerate many of these drugs without having it interfere with your weight loss efforts. When I work with patients who suffer from Bipolar disorder, I involve their psychiatrist early in the process to ensure that we optimize these medications to a more weight neutral regimen without compromising their mood stability. Bipolar disorder is a debilitating condition that can result in significant compromise of a patient's quality of life. Often, we decide that it is more important to stay on medications despite their weight gaining effects to ensure that they remain emotionally stable and maintain their relationships with their family and friends. If we can optimize other factors, we may be able to partially counteract the weight gaining effects of the medication and maintain adequate treatment of their mood disorder.

Chronic Pain and Neuropathy Medications: The two most common medications used for treating these conditions are Neurontin® (Gabapentin) and Lyrica® (Pregablin). Chronic Pain and Neuropathy are complicated conditions that offer many options for non-pharmacologic treatment; including exercise, meditation, and nutrition. I work with patients who are on these medications to ensure that we optimize all other treatment options in an effort to eliminate or decrease the dose of these two medications. As with all the other medications we've discussed, I ensure that the prescribing physician has the final say.

Insulin: There is a distinct crossroads in the health of any patient who suffers from diabetes that occurs the moment their physician discusses starting insulin. Diabetes is a disease that is at least partially caused by a reaction to our processed, Western diet and is tightly linked to obesity. Unfortunately, Insulin, our most effective treatment for the elevated blood sugar that occurs as a result of diabetes, is also a potent fat storage medication[30]. Most patients who start on insulin will gain 20-30 pounds. The result is that even though their blood sugars improve, the insulin induced weight gain worsens the underlying disease– they respond less and less to the insulin that their body makes and that they inject. A dangerous spiral ensues as the dose of insulin is increased to overcome the increased insulin resistance, causing even more weight gain and further decreasing their body's ability to respond to insulin.

For years, I have encouraged primary care physicians and endocrinologists to present patients at this difficult crossroads in the progression of their diabetes with an option to start a course of intense nutritional intervention and have an evaluation for bariatric surgery. For some, nutritional modification alone is all that is necessary to prevent the need for insulin. Others may require bariatric surgery which will stop the spiral immediately and usually put patients' diabetes into complete remission.

Sleep Medications: A lack of sleep can be a major contributor to weight gain, but you also have to watch out for medications that are meant to help you sleep better. Thankfully, most sleep medications are not concerning, however, there is a class that can cause weight gain. Trazodone[31] and Risperidone[32] are medications that have powerful sedating effects that make them very effective sleep-inducing agents. Unfortunately, they also cause significant weight gain. If weight is a concern, you should avoid the use of these medications.

This list is partial and merely represents the most common weight gaining medications that I see in my practice. There are many others that can cause weight gain as well as a number of medications that most people believe cause weight gain that often don't. Most antidepressants[33] and oral contraceptives[34] do not cause significant weight gain, despite popular opinion. Also, most medications that target your cardiovascular system or digestive tract do not impact your weight. Again, please consult with your physician before adjusting the dose of any of these medications or stopping them outright. I always work closely with the prescribing physicians and leave the final decision about a particular medication up to the physician and patient to discuss separately.

Inactivity and Injury

A prolonged period of inactivity- whether it is caused by an injury or by life factors like work, school, or personal demands- typically results in a loss of muscle mass. One critical factor in determining your metabolic thermostat's set point is the amount of healthy muscle that you have[35]. Building muscle is difficult and losing it is easy. Even a few days of a sedentary lifestyle in a previously active adult can result in decreased strength and loss of muscle. Inactivity and injury are very common causes of weight gain in my practice. I've heard many, many stories of patients who were a few pounds overweight, but remained active until they injured their back or knee, or suffered some other injury that prevented them from maintaining their active lifestyle. These injuries can result in 40-50 pounds of weight gain that is often irreversible.

Another way that injury can cause weight gain is by blocking the functionality of the overfed side of your metabolic thermostat. When you gain those first few pounds, a functional metabolic thermostat will result in an increase in your metabolism and you will (subconsciously) be more willing to walk faster, take the stairs, go to the gym, or perform any other activities that will burn more calories[36]. However, if every time you stand up to move, you experience pain from your injury, your ability to upregulate your metabolism through additional movement is compromised. Factors that impede the proper functioning of the overfed side of your metabolic thermostat can result in an often-permanent increase in your set point.

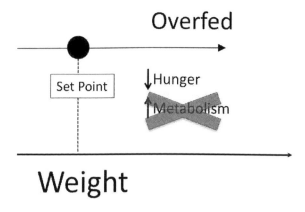

Figure 3 - An injury prevents your metabolic rate from increasing

Food Addictions

Most of the foods available in our nation's grocery stores are heavily processed. Our food supply has become so distorted that the idea of avoiding foods that are made in a manufacturing plant seems nearly impossible. Processed foods are the creation of food chemists- not chefs. Becoming a food chemist requires a college degree as well as a significant amount of training afterward. Food chemists experiment with combinations of flours, oils, sugars, flavorings, and sweeteners to create "foodstuff" that is relatively non-perishable, irresistible, and inexpensive to make. They then take their creations and test them against a focus group to ensure that everyone finds their foods as irresistible as possible. If the focus group isn't instantly hooked, it's back to the lab to make adjustments until they are.

As a result of their brilliant food chemistry, we as a nation have become completely addicted to processed foods. These foods trigger the pleasure centers of our brain the same way that alcohol, drugs, and tobacco do[37]. As a result, many of us have become completely addicted. Food addictions are very real and cause us to eat in the absence of hunger. Eating in order to feed an addiction, rather than to address hunger also disrupts the functioning of the overfed side of your metabolic thermostat.

If you gain a few pounds and shift toward the overfed side of your metabolic thermostat, you will have less hunger and less of a desire to eat. However, if you are addicted to certain high calorie foods, you will eat even when you are not hungry. Food addictions derail the overfed side of your metabolic thermostat; sabotaging your body's attempts to maintain a stable weight. The only way to combat food addictions is to treat them the same way that we treat addictions to alcohol, tobacco, or drugs and to avoid these substances altogether. There also may be a role for some weight loss medications that help with food addictions that we'll detail in the next chapter.

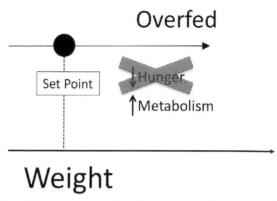

Weight

Figure 4 – Addiction to processed foods prevents your hunger from decreasing

Sugar Sweetened Beverages

In my opinion, these are the most fattening "foods" on the planet. We all think about soda as the worst culprit, but there are many other beverages that are just as bad. Many people fail to realize that fruit juices (all of them) contain nearly as much sugar as soda and are nearly as dangerous. Other offending beverages include sports drinks like Gatorade or Powerade, energy drinks like Monster or Red Bull, sweetened coffee drinks, sugar in your coffee, sweet tea, lemonade, and Kool-Aid.

Most people point to the fact that sugar sweetened beverages are empty calories that contain tons of sugar as the reason they should be avoided. However, their true danger is much subtler and more sinister. Our body has a complicated system that regulates thirst and a separate one that manages hunger. There is little to no crossover between the two systems. We understand this intuitively. Drinking a glass of water does little to satisfy your hunger and eating a steak will not make you less thirsty. When we drink a sugar sweetened beverage, it is tallied in the thirst column- not the hunger column. Drinking a sugar sweetened beverage does nothing to reduce your hunger. Because sweetened beverages are viewed as liquids that reduce thirst rather than food that addresses hunger, the calories they contain do not alter your metabolic thermostat and do nothing to reduce hunger or the amount of food that you subsequently consume. The ability to consume calories without it resulting in a decrease in your hunger is the perfect recipe for weight gain[38].

Because our metabolic thermostat is always functioning to adjust our hunger and metabolic rate, we are very good at matching the calories we consume to those that we burn. We all know people who weigh the same amount that they did 20 years ago. These people have such a highly functioning thermostat that they've been able to balance their calorie consumption and calorie expenditure down to the last crumb. Assuming that you need to store 3,500 calories to create one pound of body fat, converting 10 calories a day into fat every day for 20 years will result in more than 20 pounds of weight gain. So, if you weigh the same as you did 20 years ago, you must have burned exactly the same number of calories that you've consumed, down to the last crumb. Over twenty years, this is a remarkable task that could never be accomplished through discipline or willpower. It can only be accomplished through tight physiologic regulation.

If you are consuming sugar sweetened beverages on a regular basis, you are consistently delivering calories that are not considered by your metabolic thermostat. Because the sugar is delivered in liquid form, our brain focuses on the liquid- not the calories. You'll be less thirsty after downing a soft drink, but not less hungry. This has been demonstrated in studies that measure food consumption patterns after ingesting calories in either liquid or solid form[38,39]. Calories consumed in solid form will decrease subsequent food consumption. Your metabolic thermostat recognizes the calories in the solid food and you subconsciously eat less throughout the remainder of the day. Calories consumed in liquid form do not result in the same adjustment of future calorie consumption since your metabolic thermostat does not respond appropriately to liquid calories.

Drinking just one 12-ounce sugar sweetened beverage per day has the potential to increase your storage of calories to the tune of 15 pounds per year[i]. We often rationalize the comparatively low number of calories in these beverages in comparison to the total number of calories that we consume each day. However, calories in liquid form are not equal to those in solid form. Step number one of any weight loss plan (surgical or non-surgical) must be to immediately eliminate all sugar sweetened beverages from your diet. Many people report headaches or withdrawal symptoms once they stop drinking sugar sweetened beverages. However, it's usually not the absence of sugar that is causing the symptoms, it's the absence of caffeine. If you replace the caffeine that you were consuming in the sugary drink, it's much easier to eliminate sugar sweetened beverages from your diet. Substituting your caffeinated, sugar sweetened beverage with coffee (without sugar), un-sweet tea (iced or warm), or even caffeinated water (there are several brands available), will allow you to eliminate these potent set point elevating beverages from your life once and for all.

Yo-Yo Dieting

As you are starting to learn, it is impossible to fight your physiology in your efforts to lose weight. Yo-yo dieting is a **temporary** change in the *quantity* of calories you consume, rather than what is required for durable weight loss – a **permanent** change in the *quality* of the calories you consume (more on this later). If your focus is to decrease your calorie consumption through smaller portion sizes, choosing heavily processed low calorie or low-fat foods, or by replacing meals with low calorie shakes or frozen foods, you are setting yourself up for an unwinnable war against your physiology. Your body will not view your new meal plan the same way you do. It will view it as a famine. Your metabolic thermostat does not consider the

---

[i] Assuming the 12 ounce beverage contains 150 calories

intentions of your weight loss efforts- just the impact of fewer calories. Even if your blood pressure and cholesterol levels are high and your physician tells you that you're showing early signs of diabetes, your body is not able to recognize that this calorie restriction will improve your health.

The result of your self-imposed starvation will be the hunger and metabolic changes that we discussed in the last chapter. Your hunger will increase and your metabolism will slow, sabotaging your ability to stick to your diet or exercise program. The result is inevitable. Once you resume your normal eating pattern while your metabolic thermostat is in starvation mode you will rapidly regain all of the weight you've lost and often a few extra few pounds for good measure. Yo-yo dieting (known as weight cycling in the medical literature) often results in a net weight gain as your body gradually shifts more toward a fat storage mode as a result of the frequent, random periods of starvation you impose[40]. Yo-yo dieting has also been shown to increase cardiovascular risk factors and even mortality[41]. Weight loss does not have to be painful- despite popular opinion. As we will discuss in detail later, there are much more sensible ways to lose weight than by imposing temporary periods of starvation.

Genetics

We all know someone who never gains weight despite eating large amounts of processed foods. If you are reading this book, chances are that you are not one of them. Our physiology evolved in an environment in which food was scarce and our metabolic thermostat worked to ensure that we made the most of the calories we were able to consume. There is a wide variation in the efficiency of our fat storage capabilities[42]. Some people are very efficient at storing their excess calories as body fat, while others are resistant to fat storage. Ten thousand years ago, an efficient fat storage physiology was an advantage and allowed some cavemen to make it through the winter with ease while others were on the brink of starvation. This "improved" physiology is now a disadvantage in our food abundant modern environment.

Obesity is not a fair and equitable disease. Yes, your diet absolutely impacts your body weight. However, the way your body manages these calories is even more important. For many, eating a small amount of processed food daily will result in weight gain, while others are able to eat a predominantly processed food diet and not gain weight. Your resistance to the weight gaining effects of processed food is the result of your genetics, your environment as a developing fetus, your childhood diet, and your life experiences. We are only beginning to understand the science behind these important differences between thin people and those who suffer from obesity. Our societal view of obesity has a long way to go before we, as a community, recognize obesity as an unfair disease and that those who suffer are victims-not weak-minded individuals who are unable to control their appetite.

The wonderful thing about weight loss surgery is that it offers you a chance at another ticket in the fat storage lottery. The results after surgery vary significantly from individual to individual[43]. Some post-surgical patients become highly resistant to the weight gaining effects of processed foods despite decades of living with a powerful fat storing metabolism. Others are able to lose the weight initially but remain highly susceptible to weight regain from processed foods. This critical point will be discussed in much more detail in later chapters.

Pregnancy and Menopause

Weight gain during pregnancy is expected and the failure of any pregnant woman to gain weight during a pregnancy is cause for concern. However, coupling our food abundant modern environment with an "eating for two" philosophy is a recipe for disaster for many women. When I work with women of childbearing age and discuss plans for pregnancy, I make the point that these nine months are the most critical time in your life to follow a healthy eating plan. Because your body will naturally increase your set point, it is critical to avoid processed foods and inactivity to ensure that your set point does not increase beyond the 20-30 pounds that it needs to support a healthy pregnancy. After delivery, your hormonal state will return to normal and your set point usually returns to within a few pounds of your pre-pregnancy weight. However, if you fan the flames of your pregnancy induced set point elevation by eating large amounts of processed, calorie dense foods, the additional weight gain caused by the processed foods may not be corrected after your body returns to its normal hormonal state.

Furthermore, the "eating for two" advice given to pregnant women must be adapted in response to our increased understanding of the causes of obesity. These nine months are not only critical to your own future body weight, they will also strongly impact your child's health. A healthy or unhealthy maternal diet will significantly alter a fetus's in-utero environment and will play a critical role in that child's future relationship with food and tendency to gain weight[44].

Menopause also results in set point elevation in many women. While most women gain only five to ten pounds from the hormonal changes of menopause, some can gain 30 pounds or even more. In my experience, postmenopausal women, as a group, have the most difficult time losing weight when we opt for non-surgical treatment programs. Menopause can cause a significant change in your fat storage metabolism making you very resistant to using nutritional means to achieve weight loss[45]. However, I have not found menopause to be a significant obstacle to weight loss after surgery. I am usually quick to recommend adding surgery to a postmenopausal woman's weight loss treatment plan.

Stress and Depression

There is a very tight link between stress, depression, and obesity. It's very difficult to determine whether stress and depression cause obesity or whether obesity causes stress and depression. It's likely that both are true, creating a dangerous cycle of positive feedback. Stress and depression cause weight gain, which in turn, causes increased stress and depression.

Our body's response to stress in our modern environment is quite different from the stress response that our ancestors experienced. For cavemen, acute stress was of primary concern. Our primal environment was ripe with thousands of potentially deadly encounters. There were no guardrails on the edge of the cliff and the mountain lions and grizzly bears were not penned up in a cage in the zoo. They roamed freely, possibly around the next bend. Our physiology is extremely effective at dealing with these acutely stressful threats. If you walk out of your cave and find yourself staring right into the eyes of a mountain lion, our stress response system will cause your pupils to dilate, your muscles will tighten, your heart will speed up, and you will be able to run faster, jump higher, and fight harder than you ever thought you could.

Fortunately, acute danger is relatively rare in our modern environment. However, financial concerns, marital strain, and stress in your workplace often pervade our daily life. We don't have a separate system for dealing with chronically stressful situations, so we use the only one we have and try to approach our child's bad report card the same way our ancestors dealt with dangerous mountain lions. The result is the over release of cortisol and several other chemicals that can shift our body toward fat storage[46].

Successful weight loss (with or without the use of surgery) is dependent on developing better methods of handling the chronic stress that all of us deal with. While there is no shortage of anti-depressants and anti-anxiety medications, they rarely result in significant improvements. On the other hand, exercise, meditation, exposure to nature and counselling are often truly helpful ways to reduce the amount of stress or sadness in your life. Exploring all possible options is critical to ensure that we've done our best to reduce the weight gaining effects of untreated stress or depression.

Altered Sleep

People who work the night shift often have an exceptionally difficult time losing weight[47]. In our 24-hour modern economy, a significant percentage of us work at night and sleep during the day. This pattern goes directly against our natural circadian rhythms. It alters our eating patterns and often results in significantly less sleep and lower quality sleep than those of us who keep a more traditional schedule.

This disrupted sleep is even more problematic when people cycle back and forth from nighttime sleep to daytime sleep frequently. This often occurs when night shift workers change back to a daytime schedule during their time off so they can spend time with family and friends. The constant shift from sleeping during the day to sleeping at night alters your metabolism and your appetite.

Many people think that the weight gain is due to eating a more processed diet since it's hard to get a good salad at 3am, but this is only part of the problem. A dysregulation of your sleep/wake cycle slows down your metabolism and increases your hunger – the exact effects seen when your metabolic thermostat's set point is increased.

Unfortunately, many people are dependent on night shift hours for their job, family or financial stability. It may not be reasonable to shift to a daytime schedule in order to meet your weight loss goals. Working the night shift does not make it impossible to lose weight, it just makes it much more difficult.

Other Causes

The above discussion does not represent a comprehensive list of the causes of set point elevation, only those that I see most often in my practice. Other factors like chronic disease and hormones found in beef can also contribute to increasing your body's set point but are typically minor factors.

One common point of confusion is the belief that eliminating the things that make your set point to go up will cause your weight to go down. Unfortunately, when you eliminate the medications, processed foods, and sugar sweetened beverages from your diet, you usually don't lose weight[48]. Instead, you just stop gaining weight. Most consumers of sugar sweetened beverages can attest to this. In most cases, stopping the soda results in no more than a few pounds of weight loss. This is often cited as an excuse to continue drinking the sugary beverages. I have heard many patients tell me that they stopped drinking soda in the past and didn't lose weight so they figured that it must not be the cause of their obesity.

Before you're able to lose weight, you must eliminate those things in your life that are causing your set point to go up. However, lowering your set point requires a different set of changes from those discussed above. In the next chapter, we'll discuss the four ways that you can lower your set point.

CHAPTER FOUR
HOW TO LOSE WEIGHT

There are four ways to lower your set point. We will explore them all in detail, however, the remainder of the book will focus on the final and most effective method- weight loss surgery. When you lower your set point, your body will view your current weight as lying on the overfed side of your metabolic thermostat and will trigger your hunger to decrease and your metabolism to increase. You will effortlessly shed pounds until your weight matches your new lower set point. Again, this is the holy grail of weight loss since your physiology is now driving you to decrease your fat stores, rather than fighting against it.

Let's review the four ways that you can lower your set point:

1. A change in the quality of your diet

2. Building muscle and using it

3. Medications

4. Weight loss surgery

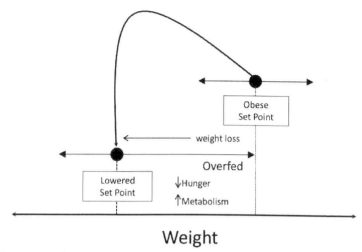

Weight

Figure 5 - A lowered set point allows you to lose weight without increased hunger or a decreased metabolic rate

A Change in the Quality of Your Diet

Changing the quality of your diet is very different than trying to lose weight by restricting your calorie intake. Most dieters believe that the act of eating causes weight gain and will direct their efforts toward trying to eat as little as possible. However, now that we understand the control your metabolic thermostat has on your hunger and metabolism, we recognize that your body views your efforts to lose weight through calorie restriction as an unwelcome period of starvation. Eating, in and of itself, is not responsible for weight gain and starving yourself will not result in durable weight loss[49].

Instead, we must look at eating in greater detail to determine the best ways to change your diet in order to drive weight loss. There are some foods that actually trigger weight loss while others trigger weight gain. The nutritional changes that result in a lowering of your set point were explained in great detail in my first book, A Pound of Cure, which can serve as a reference for those of you looking for more information about this style of eating.

Perhaps the best example of how eating more of certain foods drives weight loss is by considering the following hypothetical case. If you were to start eating three pounds of broccoli a day, but not make any other conscious changes to the way that you eat, do you think that you would lose weight or gain it? Most of us recognize that this change in your diet would very likely result in weight loss because you would eat less of the calorie dense foods that typically make up the majority of your diet.

It turns out that there are many foods that are associated with weight loss beyond green vegetables. When dietary surveys are performed across large numbers of people, we find that increased consumption of vegetables, fruit, nuts, seeds, beans, and yogurt are repeatedly found to correlate with leanness- not obesity[50,51]. While our scientific understanding of why those of us who eat more of these unprocessed foods are thinner is not clear, it is likely that the answer lies in the thousands of largely undiscovered phytonutrients that are found in abundance in a plant-based diet.

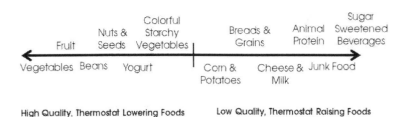

Figure 6 - The Spectrum of Food Quality

Fruits, vegetables, nuts, seeds, yogurt, and beans are all thermostat lowering, nutrient dense foods. "Nutrient Dense" means that they contain lots of nutrition in very few calories. The more of these foods you eat, the more weight you lose. Most of the foods in the average American's diet are breads, fried foods, sugar sweetened foods, and sugar sweetened beverages. These foods are highly processed, thermostat raising, and calorie dense. They contain lots of calories, but very little nutrition. Increased consumption of thermostat lowering, nutrient dense foods like vegetables tend to "crowd out" your consumption of calorie dense, thermostat raising, processed foods. The result of consuming large amounts of vegetables and other thermostat lowering, nutrient dense foods is a significant improvement in the quality of the calories that you consume- often without decreasing the quantity of calories you consume.

Improving the quality of your diet by eating primarily vegetables, fruit, nuts, seeds, yogurt, and beans results in a gradual lowering of your set point that allows you to shed a few pounds per month without feeling hungry or run down like you do on starvation diets[52]. When I work with patients trying to change their diet, I often make the point that they are 1,000 pounds of vegetables away from lowering their set point down to their goal weight. At two pounds of vegetables per day, it would take just under a year and a half to eat all 1,000 pounds. This points out the gradual, cumulative effect of a qualitative diet change on your set point.

Another concept that is often helpful as a guide to improving the quality of your diet is to consider the ratio of thermostat lowering, nutrient dense calories that you consume to those that come from thermostat raising, processed, calorie dense foods. I refer to this as your "CaloRatio." I use it as a guide to offer a numerical measurement of the quality of your diet. I've released a free smartphone app (called CaloRatio) and website (www.caloratio.com) that I use with my patients to help them measure the quality of the calories they consume.

Long ago, we separated healthy eating from eating for weight loss. This change in perspective single handedly launched the diet industry and jumpstarted the obesity epidemic. If we hope to make any progress in losing weight permanently, it is critical that we reunite the concepts of eating for health and eating for weight loss.

By counting the ratio of good calories to bad calories, rather than focusing on the total number of calories, we de-emphasize portion control and instead, focus on helping the dieter improve the quality of the food they consume. As you work to maximize your CaloRatio for the day, you will find that you respond differently to those inevitable moments that you find yourself powerless to resist the draw of an unhealthy food choice. The typical calorie counter's response to a "cheat meal" is to skip the next meal in order to ensure that your total calorie count for the day does not rise any further. Unfortunately, this is perhaps the worst reaction since it triggers your body to enter starvation mode and store that chocolate chip cookie rather than burn it. When eating to optimize your CaloRatio, eating chocolate chip cookies or other calorie dense foods can only be countered by consuming a large amount of nutrient dense, thermostat lowering food like fruits, vegetables, nuts, seeds, and beans.

Postoperative weight loss surgery patients thrive on a high CaloRatio diet. Weight loss surgery causes an immediate lowering of your set point, putting you on the extreme end of the overfed side of the spectrum[53]. This causes your body to burn off your excess fat stores to bring your body weight down to your newly lowered set point. When your body is driving you to lose weight, you will start craving fruit, vegetables, nuts, seeds, beans, and yogurt. You'll have no taste for the processed fare that most of us craved before surgery[54]. It's critical for postoperative patients to harness this redirection of your taste preferences by creating new habits and new personal philosophies about food. Your ability to do this successfully over the first 1-2 years after surgery is one of the most important factors that will contribute to your long-term postoperative success.

Building Muscle and Using It

The majority of us who exercise in an effort to lose weight select low intensity, cardiovascular activities like the treadmill, elliptical, or stationary bike. While these are helpful for improving your heart and lung health, they do little to drive meaningful weight loss[55,56]. Now that we understand the importance of our metabolic thermostat's set point in our weight loss efforts, we have to take another look at exercise.

When considering exercise, the most important factor that influences our metabolic thermostat's set point is the amount of healthy muscle that we have[35,57]. **Exercising to achieve weight loss should focus on movements that work to build muscle instead of those that work to burn calories.** The weight loss effects of muscle building exercises are evident if you pay close attention the next time you walk through your local gym. The weight room is typically filled with well-developed lean men and women while the treadmill and elliptical room houses those who are struggling to lose weight. Because we've been obsessed with calorie balance as the primary determinant of weight loss for so many years, we bought into the idea of low intensity movement, performed for long periods of time, as the best form of exercise for weight loss. We've always believed that the longer you stay on the treadmill, elliptical, or Stairmaster, the more weight you will lose.

Now that we are viewing obesity as an elevation in our set point, rather than an unfavorable tipping of our calorie balance, low intensity exercises like the elliptical, treadmill, or Stairmaster no longer make sense as the optimal exercise regimen. Instead, we must look to higher intensity exercises, performed for a short period of time (typically 20 minutes or less), if we are going to use exercise to drive permanent, set point lowering weight loss. Exercising to build muscle is primarily dependent on the *intensity* of the movements, rather than the *duration* that you perform them for[58,59]. This critical paradigm shift requires us to completely rethink our workout.

High intensity exercise is not for everyone and must be implemented carefully under the guidance of your physician and an experienced personal trainer. I've found exercise to be an extremely useful weight loss tool for women under 30 and men under 40 years old. As you age, your ability to build muscle decreases, and the likelihood that you suffer from orthopedic problems increases, making high intensity exercise less effective and more dangerous.

Whatever exercise methodology you decide on, it is absolutely critical that you do everything within your power to decrease your chances of injury. As we discussed previously, an injury that results in a prolonged period of inactivity can result in significant- often irreversible- weight gain. The goal of your exercise plan is to improve your health and lower your set point. If you're not careful and perform a workout that is beyond your physical capabilities, the opposite can occur. Another critical component of injury prevention is to use proper form when exercising. Selecting weights that are too heavy will prevent you from using proper form. Exercising to the point of injury will cause weight gain and decreased fitness, exactly the opposite of what you are tyring to achieve.

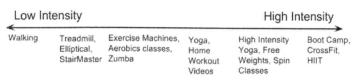

Figure 7- The spectrum of exercise intensity

Just as there is a nutritional spectrum for lowering your thermostat with foods, a similar spectrum exists for exercise. Your goal is to select the most intense exercise that you're capable of performing safely. Younger patients, without orthopedic limitations, should consider high intensity yoga, free weights, spin classes as well as boot camp, CrossFit, and other High Intensity Interval Training (HIIT) workouts. HIIT drives you to work out at a near maximal intensity for short time periods. Think sprinting uphill for a minute or doing as many push-ups in a row as you can until you collapse from exhaustion. After a short interval of high intensity, you can rest for a minute or so before you jump right back into another high intensity interval. Typically, 20-30 minutes of these intervals are all you need to increase your fitness and drive weight loss[60,61]. While this is a welcome change from 60 minutes on the treadmill, 15 minutes of HIIT can sometimes feel like an hour.

Those patients who are older, or suffer from orthopedic limitations, should select workouts from the lower intensity side of the spectrum like walking outside, using an elliptical or treadmill, the Stairmaster, Zumba or aerobics classes, or weight machines. However, even if you are limited by your age, low level of fitness, or orthopedic injuries, with a little patience you can usually work your way up to be able to participate in yoga classes. Yoga offers particular advantages over other lower intensity exercise techniques. First, it works more to increase your muscle strength than other low intensity forms of exercise. Second, it is one of the safest forms of exercise when performed properly and can help you increase your flexibility. Improved flexibility is vital to future injury prevention. Finally, it offers a guiding philosophy that enthusiasts find helpful in managing stress which we've already described as a contributor to weight gain.

In fact, exercise may be the single best treatment for chronic stress. Medications are largely ineffective and indulging in food, alcohol, drugs, or tobacco typically worsen stress in the long run, rather than relieve it. I always challenge patients who are having difficulty meeting their weight loss goals due to chronic stress to adopt an exercise program. Even low intensity exercise offers tremendous stress relief[62]. There are very few problems that aren't improved by 30 minutes of exercise.

The most important reason to exercise is not for assistance in weight loss. In fact, as we age, exercise alone results in very minimal weight loss[63]. And, while younger people are able to succeed using high intensity workouts, this weight loss is typically short lived unless it's also accompanied by significant nutritional changes as well[64]. Patients who rely on exercise as their primary mode of weight loss are one injury away from regaining every pound. So, if this is true, why should we bother with exercise at all? **The primary reason that we should exercise is not to drive weight loss, but to help maintain our weight loss over the long run[65,66].**

Medications

Now that we are looking at weight loss with a new understanding of our metabolic thermostat's role in regulating our fat stores, it seems entirely possible that medications could influence your body's set point. As we've discussed, there are many medications that adjust your set point upward, so it makes sense that there must be some that adjust it downward. Unfortunately, when we look closely at the weight loss medications that are currently available, we find that a "miracle drug" simply does not exist. While it is entirely possible, and even probable, that this medication will be developed within the next 25 years, it has not been developed yet and there are no realistic candidates in the research pipeline at this time.

Most physicians who prescribe weight loss medications reserve them for use only after nutritional changes and exercise have been implemented. There is wide variation in the response rate to weight loss medications[67,68]. While most people do not achieve significant weight loss, there is a distinct subset that can lose and maintain 10% of their body weight with the right medication regimen. However, the effect is only maintained for as long as you are taking the medication. Now that we understand the impact of our metabolic thermostat on our hunger and metabolic rate, and the role of medications in lowering our body's set point, this is a natural conclusion. When you stop taking the set point lowering medication, your set point drifts back up and you will regain weight. In most circumstances, lifelong use of weight loss medications is required if the weight loss is to be maintained.

These limitations make medications a very small part of my therapeutic approach to treating patients for obesity without surgery. However, weight loss medications can be very helpful if administered after surgery[69]. Often, medications can help patients who are struggling to succeed by enhancing the effect of the surgery. I do not use them on every postoperative patient; only those whose weight loss is less than what we would expect.

The most commonly used weight loss medication is Phentermine, also known as Adipex®. Adipex® has been in use since the early 70's and can trigger significant weight loss in some people. It is a stimulant drug in the amphetamine class, however, it's primary mechanism of action is to decrease your appetite rather than increase your metabolic rate[70]. Weight loss on Adipex® is typically easy without requiring a significant change in your diet. Adipex's® side effect profile prevents it from being taken indefinitely and it needs to be cycled on and off every few months. The very predictable result of this dosing pattern is a cycle of yo-yo weight loss and weight gain. Also, the effects of Adipex® may diminish over time so that patients who were initially successful with the drug, no longer see the same results the next time they start taking it[71].

Another commonly used medication is Topiramate; more commonly referred to as Topamax®. Topamax® is primarily used as an anti-seizure drug. It has some mood stabilizing effects, as well, and may be useful in treating Bipolar disorder. A pleasant side effect of Topamax® is weight loss, however it is usually limited to 5-10 pounds[72]. It typically does not cause as much weight loss as Adipex® and often does not induce any weight loss at all. But it has a very favorable side effect profile and is inexpensive, making it a popular choice. Often, Adipex® and Topamax® are used in combination. In fact, a very smart pharmaceutical executive recognized that he could patent a "new weight loss drug" that consisted of both medications in one pill. The result is Qsymia®, which has been aggressively marketed by its manufacturer[73], but has not been widely adopted by physicians or patients.

Contrave® is another example of the pharmaceutical industry using two older medications in combination as a "new drug." Contrave® contains both Bupropion (Wellbutrin®) and Naltrexone; a drug that works to block some of the pleasure signals in the brain. These two drugs in combination offer modest weight loss for a subset of patients but have very few side effects. It is brilliantly named to suggest that it reduces your cravings for food, but the science to support reduced food cravings while taking Contrave® is controversial[74]. Contrave®, like most other weight loss medications, offers variable results[67] and must also be paired with good nutrition and exercise. The average weight loss attributable to Contrave® over one year is only 5-10 pounds.

Belviq® (Lorcaserin) is a new medication that is similar to Fenfluramine, a medication that was removed from the market due to dangerous side effects[75]. Fenfluramine was once part of the popular combination drug Fen-Phen (Phentermine and fenfluramine). Fen-Phen® was pulled from the market early this century and has resulted in legal damages to the manufacturer that exceeded $13 billion dollars as a result of the class action lawsuits that followed. It appears that the manufacturers covered up fatal heart valve abnormalities attributed to the medication in early studies. Belviq® reports a much lower affinity for heart valves than was observed in fenfluramine, so there is reason to be optimistic that it won't cause the same devastating complications that we saw with fenfluramine. I rarely prescribe Belviq® due to my concerns about its safety and the modest weight loss it offers.

A recently approved weight loss medication (Dec 2014) is Saxenda® (Liraglutide). Liraglutide is also marketed under the trade name Victoza® as an injectable diabetes drug in the GLP-1 analog class. These medications have been very helpful in the treatment of diabetes and add an extra medication that can be used to help keep patients off insulin. Insulin often causes significant weight gain, while Victoza® often helps with weight loss[76].

Liraglutide (at a higher dose than Victoza®) has been re-branded for weight loss. Saxenda® is without question, the most effective weight loss medication on the market today. Despite its effectiveness, there are a few limitations to Saxenda®. The first is that it can only be taken as a daily injection. As we discussed earlier, long term success with weight loss medications requires long term use. So, any weight lost through the use of Saxenda® often commits the patient to daily injections for years to come. The second is that it can cause significant nausea and vomiting, especially within the first few weeks. When starting Saxenda®, you must start at a low dose and gradually increase the amount you inject over a month or so to get to the full, effective dose. Finally, Saxenda® is extremely expensive, often costing more than $1,000 per month[77]. While some insurance plans will cover it, many do not.

When we look closely at the weight loss medication options currently available, it is easy to explain why only 2% of the patients who qualify for a weight loss medication receive a prescription[78]. These medications are not new, despite the publicity and are only modestly effective in a subset of patients.

Bariatric Surgery

The final, and most effective, way to lower your metabolic thermostat's set point is through bariatric surgery[53]. For decades, we believed that bariatric surgery worked by preventing you from eating large portions (we refer to this as restriction) while blocking your intestines from absorbing calories (malabsorption). However, as the science of bariatric surgery grows, we are beginning to recognize that the primary way that these surgeries work is by adjusting the hormonal relationship between your brain and your gut to trigger a lowering of your set point. While restriction and malabsorption do play a role early after the surgery, the dominant effects over the long run are the hormonal, set point lowering changes[79,80,81].

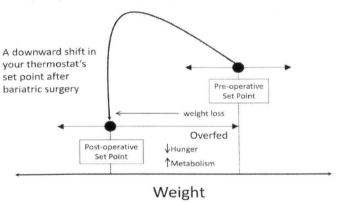

Figure 8 - Set point lowering effects of Bariatric Surgery

Examining the figure above demonstrates how bariatric surgery can trigger patients to lose their hunger and shed weight easily for an entire year after surgery. Bariatric surgery causes an immediate and significant lowering of your set point- almost overnight[82]. Within days of your surgery, your metabolic thermostat's setting will drop to your future postoperative weight, leaving a huge discrepancy between your current body weight and the weight your brain believes you should be (your new, lowered set point). This leaves your metabolism well on the "overfed" side which causes your brain, gut, and fat cells to look at your current level of fat stores as excessive. Thus, your hunger decreases and your metabolic rate increases.

I see the effects of this favorable metabolic state every day in my office. First, I see patients fail to experience significant hunger for 1-2 years after surgery. Most patient's hunger only returns after their actual body weight reaches their new, lower metabolic thermostat's setting[83]. Second, I see the subtle signs of an increased metabolism in their every movement. Patients develop a gait that I refer to as a "Gastric Bypass swagger" in which their arm, hip and leg movements become exaggerated in their body's effort to burn as many calories as possible with each stride[84].

If you examine the life of a patient after bariatric surgery closely, the impact of the metabolic effects of the surgery become clear. If the primary mechanism of weight loss was through restriction, patients would begin to regain weight once their portion sizes increase (1-2 years after surgery). But this does not occur after surgery unless the postoperative patient resumes a diet of calorie dense junk foods- or even worse- sugar sweetened beverages. If the primary mechanism of weight loss was through malabsorption, we would see patients reporting diarrhea after surgery and an examination of their stool would demonstrate undigested food. But patients don't develop diarrhea after surgery unless they make poor food choices that are either greasy or excessively sugary.

It is only by examining weight loss after bariatric surgery as the result of an immediate lowering of your set point that we can begin to understand what life after surgery is really like. **When we view weight loss surgery over the long term, the hormonal impact of the surgery is the dominant effect that we must work to maintain[85].** There is so much myth and lore surrounding weight loss surgery that is driven by our poor understanding of how these surgeries actually work. Because we have attributed weight loss after surgery to restriction and malabsorption, we have encouraged patients to "eat your protein first" to ensure that they stay well-nourished in an attempt to overcome their body's impaired ability to absorb calories. But, ten years after Gastric Bypass surgery, the predominant problem is weight regain[86]- not starvation and a protein first mantra (especially animal protein first) may not be the ideal diet for weight loss and weight maintenance[87]. We've also encouraged patients to "avoid eating and drinking at the same time" and "avoid carbonation" for fear of stretching out their pouch and destroying the restrictive effects of the surgery. However, we see portion sizes increase in nearly all postoperative patients a few years after surgery. Yet most do not regain a significant amount of weight[88].

Now that we are looking at bariatric surgery as a set point lowering surgery, not a restrictive and malabsorptive one, the rules for success after surgery change dramatically. The remainder of this book will re-examine Bariatric Surgery taking our improved understanding of the actual mechanism of weight loss, hormonal changes, into consideration.

CHAPTER FIVE
SHOULD I HAVE WEIGHT LOSS SURGERY?

To fully examine the question of whether or not you should have weight loss surgery, we must first rephrase the question. The actual question that you should ask yourself is: Can I lower my set point by modifying my diet and increasing my exercise, or is surgery the only treatment that will work? When we examine this question, we are able to abandon the unhelpful, self-esteem depleting view of surgery as "the easy way out," or "cheating." Most patients have convinced themselves that if they could just improve their willpower, they could lose the weight and keep it off. In my mind, the willpower argument is useless and only results in shame, guilt and depression. Willpower is rarely the missing ingredient in achieving success. What is missing is an accurate understanding of obesity and how weight loss surgery works. Once we develop an understanding of our metabolic thermostat and the role of surgery, nutrition and exercise in adjusting our thermostat, we are able to make sensible decisions about our options for weight loss that are based on physiology and devoid of useless, self-defeating, emotional condemnations.

In my practice, I treat all patients who suffer from obesity, not just those who have chosen to undergo bariatric surgery. I see patients at all points in the decision-making process, from those who have no interest in having surgery to those who are eager to schedule their surgery as soon as possible. Often, I find that my assessment of whether or not a patient truly **needs** bariatric surgery in order to lose weight differs from their own opinions and I will work with these patients for several months before we come to a joint decision. Often, I find that I'm able to show the eager surgical patient that by implementing my Pound of Cure nutritional program, they can meet their weight loss and health goals without surgery. Just as often, I work with patients who are not interested in surgery initially, but after months of good compliance with the Pound of Cure program recognize that their set point is tightly fixed, and their weight loss and health goals can only be achieved through surgery. Again, surgery should be used for the patient who is unable to lose weight despite making significant nutritional changes, not the patient who is unable to make these changes in the first place.

Every patient is different and there are no hard and fast rules that allow me to determine whether surgery is necessary at their first appointment. Instead, I find that after 3-6 months of working together, we are usually able to come to the same conclusion about surgery. Despite our extremely low complication rate and high success rate with surgery, it's important to recognize that meeting your goals without a trip to the operating room is the best possible outcome. Just as importantly, it's critical that we recognize that not everyone is capable of achieving weight loss through nutritional modification and exercise alone. Contrary to popular opinion, a change in your diet does not trigger long term, sustained weight loss in everyone. I have worked with hundreds of patients who are only able to lose a few pounds despite making significant improvements in their diet.

Most people have been convinced by the media, their physicians and their skinny friends that if they just managed to get their eating under control, their weight problem would disappear. Unfortunately, for a large group of people, the physiology of our metabolic thermostat makes sustained, permanent weight loss through dieting alone impossible[89,90]. The cumulative effects of their genetics, past life experiences and current health all conspire to maintain a tightly fixed set point that will not respond to changes in their diet or increases in their level of exercise.

In order to determine whether a patient truly needs surgery, I ease my patients into our Pound of Cure nutritional program over a period of a few months and look for two results. First, I want to see if they lose weight easily and steadily, month after month. I look for a minimum weight loss of 2% of their total body weight each month, however 3-4% per month is ideal, especially in the first few months. I also like to see the patient move steadily past the 10% total body weight loss mark without slowing down. If you are not moving your set point and only losing weight because of decreased calorie consumption, you will typically plateau after losing 10% of your total body weight[15]. It is at this point that your hunger increases and your metabolism slows down to the point where further weight loss becomes extremely difficult. When I see patients losing beyond the 10% mark and not reporting significant hunger or food cravings on the Pound of Cure program, I look at this as the result of a lowered set point, making me question the necessity of surgery to achieve the same goal.

The second factor that I look for in patients who I believe will be able to succeed without surgery is that they enjoy following our Pound of Cure program and find it easy to fit this new way of eating into their lifestyle. Long term weight loss success requires long term dietary change and if you are miserable on the Pound of Cure plan, then the chances that you will continue to adhere to it for the rest of your life are exceedingly small. The patients who are likely to avoid the need for surgery are those who enjoy eating large portions of fruits and vegetables. I also use their ability to comply with the Pound of Cure program when I discuss procedure choice with patients, but we'll leave the details of this discussion for later.

As important as your enjoyment of your new, healthier diet is the absence of hunger. When you switch from a diet of largely processed foods to one that primarily consists of plants, your total, daily calorie consumption usually (but not always) decreases. If you find that your cravings for processed foods do not decrease after a few months on the program and you are constantly hungry, then it is likely that we're not seeing weight loss from set point movement. We are likely seeing the same type of weight loss you experience on a reduced calorie diet. Your set point remains fixed despite your increased consumption of set point lowering foods, so each pound that you lose triggers an increase in your hunger. Your hunger and happiness are very tightly linked- those who are losing weight without experiencing hunger are typically a very happy crowd.

While a trial of our Pound of Cure program is my ultimate litmus test to determine whether or not a patient truly requires weight loss surgery to be successful, there are several other factors that I take into consideration when I counsel patients.

Age

There are very few objective measurements of a person that can more accurately predict your ability to lose weight than your age. Weight loss for those in their sixties requires a much more significant commitment than it does for those in their twenties. As we age, our muscle mass decreases which also decreases our basal metabolic rate, making it that much more difficult to lose weight. Young people are able to participate in high intensity exercise; however, this becomes much more difficult as we approach middle age. As we age, our ability to lose weight through modifications of our nutrition and exercise alone decreases.

Also, the length of time that you must maintain your weight loss varies significantly with your age. After seventy, we tend to lose weight, not gain it[91], so those in their twenties must maintain their post-surgical weight loss for forty to fifty years after surgery, while those in their sixties only need to do so for ten or fewer years. When I meet with younger patients, I typically try to dissuade them from pursuing a surgical route. The question that I pose to the younger patient who is convinced that surgery is their only option is "when should we do this?" Perhaps it would be better to wait until after you've had children or you are more settled in your career? The answer to this question is difficult and cannot be determined by anyone else - it requires you to be honest with yourself and recognize that these surgeries do not offer guarantees, only opportunities.

Weight loss surgery offers a once in a lifetime opportunity to lower your set point. This is precious and must be treasured and nurtured. It requires you to eat and live differently than most of your family and peers. If at any time, you drop your guard and join the rest of the world in their regular consumption of processed foods, you put yourself at significant risk for weight regain and set point elevation.

Most young people have a lifetime full of new experiences waiting for them including marriage, children and new professional or social opportunities. Each of these new experiences, while often exciting and joyful, will modify your relationship with food. Finding your life partner and getting married is wonderful and emotionally fulfilling, but now there is another person involved in your daily decisions about what and where to eat. Parenthood can be amazing and wondrous, but often results in an increased consumption of leftover chicken nuggets. Your new job may offer a great salary and professional satisfaction, but it may require more travel and dinner meetings. Patients who are secure with their spousal relationships, have had their children and are stable financially and professionally do not have the same uncertainty ahead of them and are much more likely to be able to commit to a lifetime of good nutrition.

Age of onset of obesity

Those of you who remember being on your first diet in middle school are much less likely to respond to nutritional and exercise modifications than those who gained most of their weight later in life. If you've spent your entire life battling your weight, there is likely something about your genetics or your early childhood development (including your environment in your mother's uterus) that has made you very susceptible to our modern environment's set point raising effects. All of us, even those who are thin acknowledge that the rules of weight gain and weight loss are not fair. Some people can eat all the sweets and processed food they like without gaining any weight, while others gain a few pounds whenever they walk by a bakery. If you are a member of the large, unfortunate group of people who gain weight very easily and have a very difficult time losing weight, and you have been this way since your childhood, then your chances of achieving sustained, permanent weight loss through diet and exercise alone are lower than those people whose weight problems started later in life[92].

This rule is especially true for those of us over 40 since we were not exposed to the highly processed diet that today's young people are. If you are under 40 and were raised on macaroni and cheese and Coke products, then you may still be able to respond to nutritional change. Today's young people were exposed to a very different nutritional childhood than any other generation in history. The long-term impact of this upbringing is unknown but is very likely to result in a lifetime of weight problems. However, the physiology of young people is much more malleable than the rest of us and it may not be too late for those raised on junk food to obtain the lifelong benefits of an unprocessed diet rich in fruit, vegetables, nuts, seeds and beans.

Success in the past

You past dieting successes may or may not be a good indicator of your ability to lose weight without surgery. If you've found it easy to lose weight in the past, but always struggled with finding an eating plan that you find enjoyable and convenient, perhaps you should focus your efforts on finding a nutritional plan that works with your lifestyle. Again, we are looking to identify whether surgery is really necessary.

If you are able to easily lose weight on an extreme starvation diet, but fail other diet plans, then surgery is a much more reasonable decision. Extreme starvation plans are not sustainable and inevitably result in significant weight regain when you return to your normal eating habits[93]. It is for this reason that I like to use the Pound of Cure nutritional plan to test my patients' ability to lose weight without surgery since it does not induce starvation and is a plan that can be sustained for long periods of time.

Mobility

Limited mobility as a result of injury or joint disease is a significant disadvantage in your efforts to lose weight without surgery. When I walk into an exam room to meet a new patient and see a cane or walker, I recognize that my chances of helping this patient meet with success without surgery just dropped significantly. As we described earlier, a loss of mobility results in a loss of muscle and muscle is a critical factor for determining your body's set point[94]. If you are faced with a permanent deficit in your mobility, weight loss surgery is likely your only option for success. Nonetheless, there are exceptions to this rule, and I've worked with several patients who have lost 75 lbs. or more through nutritional changes alone despite being dependent on a walker.

Those who are unfortunate enough to have lost all of their mobility and are dependent on motorized assist devices (as opposed to canes, walkers and conventional wheelchairs) are very risky surgical candidates. Great care should be exercised in the decision to pursue weight loss surgery in this group of patients. Patients with limited mobility are much more likely to suffer from surgical complications than the rest of us[95]. I would strongly encourage any patient who is completely immobile to pursue an aggressive pre-surgical weight loss and physical therapy program to regain as much mobility as possible before undergoing surgery.

Many patients who suffer a temporary loss of mobility after an injury will gain a lot of weight in a short period of time. If you are able to return back to a high level of activity, this weight gain may be temporary and will not require surgery. However, if the effects of the injury linger and are aggravated by your excess weight, surgery may be your best option in an effort to get out of the spiral of worsening mobility → increased weight → worsening mobility. It is critical that these patients immediately enroll in physical therapy or undergo orthopedic surgery soon after their weight loss surgery in order to restore their mobility as close to their pre-injury state as possible.

Medication use

As we discussed earlier, those of you who take medications that cause weight gain are at a major disadvantage when you try to lose weight. Many had no idea that the medications that they were prescribed were contributing to their weight gain. Others knew the risks, but the medications were so important to their health that they had no choice but to take them. If you must take weight gaining medications and there is no possibility of stopping them, then your chance of success without surgery is significantly decreased.

I see this most frequently in patients who suffer from Bipolar disorder. It often takes years to find the right combination of medications to stabilize the mood swings that damage your relationships and self-worth. Often, the price for a more stable life is paid in pounds of fat added to your body despite a reasonable diet. These patients are uniquely challenging since altering their medication regimen brings the possibility of a return of the mood swings and instability that they've worked so hard to maintain over the years. In this group of patients, I encourage them to work with their psychiatrist to optimize their regimen but urge them not to compromise their mental health in the process. Often, we decide that we must maintain an unfavorable pharmacologic regimen despite its impact on body weight. These patients often require surgery to overcome the weight gaining impact of the medications and typically lose less weight after surgery than those who don't suffer from Bipolar disorder. Nonetheless, I have operated on dozens of people who have been able to meet their weight loss goals despite taking medications that cause weight gain.

Insulin is a powerful weight gaining medication, however, if you are on a relatively low dose, you may be able to find success without surgery. Many diabetics are able to decrease their insulin requirements significantly within one or two weeks on the Pound of Cure nutritional program. As you drop your insulin dose, you free yourself from the weight gaining effects of Insulin, allowing you to lose 10-20 pounds within a month or two. Often, your improved diet and first few pounds of weight loss are enough to get you completely off insulin.

Family History

Those patients who have a strong family history of obesity often find that surgery is their only realistic means for success[96]. If it seems like most members of your family are overweight or obese, despite eating a reasonable diet, then it is likely that your genes are set to favor fat storage when exposed to our processed American diet.

The rules are not fair when it comes to weight gain. Many people can eat heavily processed diets without gaining a pound, while others with less "lean" genes eat a relatively clean diet yet gain weight easily. The reason for this difference is largely unknown, but we are starting to make progress. Several genes have now been identified that are tightly linked to obesity and we're finally putting hard science behind what we've always known: certain genes predispose their owners to a lifetime of obesity[97].

However, it's important not to become too fatalistic when we consider our genetic tendencies. Weight loss surgery offers you the opportunity to draw another ticket from the genetic lottery. Many people may have genes that favor fat storage that have plagued them their entire life, yet also possess genes that make them exceptionally receptive to the favorable hormonal changes that occur after surgery. Just as there is significant variation in people's ability to lose and maintain weight before surgery, this same variability exists after surgery. The amount of weight that is lost after surgery is variable - some patients lose nearly all of their excess weight and are able to maintain their weight loss easily for decades, while others plateau well before they reach their goal weight and then struggle with weight regain. As we delve into the reasons behind this variability, we find that success after surgery has more to do with our genes than our ability to stick to a post-operative exercise program and healthy diet[98]. In my practice, I find that approximately 15% of my postop patients resemble one of those skinny people who find it extremely easy to maintain their post-surgical weight. There is clearly something different about the way their body has responded to surgery, and the answer most likely lies in their genes.

One of the most helpful questions I can ask a patient to predict success after surgery is "Do you have a first degree relative (parent, child or sibling) that has undergone Bariatric Surgery, and, if so, how did they do?" Just as a tendency to gain weight runs in families, so does success after weight loss surgery. I am always happy to see a new patient who is a close relative of one of my more successful patients. Although most of us are quick to attribute success after surgery to discipline and willpower, the science supports a favorable genetic makeup as the most important factor.

Baseline diet

Believe it or not, I love it when new patients report to me that their diet consists of lots of fast food and sugar sweetened beverages. There is plenty of room for change in these patients and we're likely to see substantial improvement in their health and weight as we implement the Pound of Cure program. Many of these patients are able to lose a substantial amount of weight by changing their diet and never need to proceed with surgery.

On the other hand, if you already eat a very healthy diet that consists of large amounts of fruit, vegetables, nuts seeds and beans and very little processed food, then you are very unlikely to lose a lot of weight when we implement the Pound of Cure plan. **If you are significantly obese, despite eating a healthy diet, then it is likely that surgery is your only realistic option for you to meet your weight loss goals.**

If you are considering Bariatric Surgery and you feel that your diet is much worse than your friends and family, then the first step is to improve your diet, not to move forward with surgery. Lifelong success after surgery is not possible without making substantial, permanent changes to your diet. Before you commit to weight loss surgery, you must first commit to improving your diet as much as you can. If these changes result in significant weight loss, then perhaps you can meet your goals without going under the knife.

Many people will struggle to fully embrace the Pound of Cure program that limits your diet to predominantly fruit, vegetables, nuts, seeds, beans and a little bit of lean animal protein. This does not necessarily mean that they are not ready to have surgery if they're unable to fully stick to the Pound of

Cure program. The hormonal changes that Bariatric Surgery induces will help to steer your taste preferences toward the foods that make up the Pound of Cure program and away from the heavily processed and sweetened foods that most of us prefer today. After surgery, you will find it much easier to follow the program since your hormonal state will be primed for you to enjoy this way of eating[54].

It's important that we're ready and willing to accept the change in our tastes that Bariatric Surgery imposes on us and be ready to welcome these healthier foods into our new and improved lifestyle. Many patients have preconceived notions about their food preferences or their ability to change the way they eat. I hear this every day as my patients report to me "I'm not a vegetable person" or "I never really eat beans." It is absolutely critical that you recognize that your current food preferences are the result of your environment, rather than a deeply ingrained, unchangeable personality trait. For some, change is easy, while others find it more difficult. But, for all of us, change is mandatory. You will not eat the same way after surgery and you must be ready not just to eat less, but to eat differently. Your ability and willingness to change your eating habits is something that you must be honest with yourself about. The surgery will do some of the work for you, but not all of it, and if you wonder whether you are ready to change, then you should also wonder whether you are ready to move forward with surgery.

However, for those who are ready and willing to make a meaningful change to the way they eat, the surgery will help you make these changes. After surgery, you will lose your taste for processed foods like pizza, burgers, chips, breads and pasta and develop a preference for Pound of Cure friendly foods like fruit, vegetables, nuts, seeds and beans. Because of this, a willingness to change is all that is necessary for success. If you struggle to fully embrace this diet change before surgery, but honestly believe that with a little help, you could integrate it fully into your life, then weight loss surgery will give you the nudge you need to make this meaningful change.

CHAPTER SIX
WHICH SURGERY SHOULD I HAVE?

There have been nearly a dozen different weight loss surgeries that have been offered over the last fifty years. Many of these procedures have been phased out in favor of less invasive, more effective options. There is a lot of debate and discussion about the different surgical options available. These discussions are often dominated by the zealots who favor one operation over all others. The most and least successful patients tend to be the most vocal, so we are often presented with a view of the best and worst aspects of each surgery, when the chances are, your results will likely fall somewhere in the middle.

When you listen to someone's account of their experiences with Bariatric Surgery, or read an online post, it's critical that you remember that the results after surgery vary from person to person. Some patients have remarkable results after surgery and find themselves easily maintaining their weight loss for the rest of their lives, while others struggle. Some easily adapt to their new lifestyle while others find it hard to let go of old habits. The genetic, emotional, physiological and biochemical reasons behind this variation are not fully understood[99]. Even after millions of procedures, we have very few tools that help us predict who will succeed after surgery and who will not. Within the next five to ten years, I believe that we will develop blood tests or other diagnostic studies that will allow us to more accurately predict an individual patient's likelihood for success after surgery. Until then, we have to accept that your success after surgery is difficult to predict. There are some things that you can do to improve your chances, but there are many other factors that are beyond your control. We must work hard to modify factors like your post-operative diet and exercise program, but also learn to accept and love ourselves if we don't meet our weight loss goals.

I always caution my patients about making a procedure choice based on one person's experience. We all know going into Bariatric Surgery that complications and difficulties after surgery can occur. We also know that it is possible to not reach your weight loss goals or regain your weight years down the road. If you have a friend who had a great experience with a Sleeve Gastrectomy, then you may too, but you also might not. As human beings, we are very drawn to people's stories to help us make sense of confusing decisions. Following a friend or loved one through the surgery and watching their recovery and ultimate success is very comforting when you make your own decision, but it's critical that you remember that stories, both good and bad, may distract you from making your best decision.

For instance, you may have a friend who has constant nausea and abdominal pain after a Gastric Bypass procedure. You suffer from diabetes and are looking for the best surgery to get you off insulin (which is a Gastric Bypass) but are concerned after watching your friend's negative experience. However, you may be missing an important piece of the puzzle - your friend smokes and has continued to smoke after the procedure, and you have never been a smoker. Patients who smoke after a Gastric Bypass procedure often develop ulcers which cause frequent nausea and abdominal pain[100] - in my practice, I refuse to perform Gastric Bypass procedures on any patients who haven't quit smoking well before surgery and acknowledge the difficulties they will have if they start again after surgery. Although your friend has had a terrible time after her surgery and urges you not to make the same mistake, her experience is unlikely to be relevant to yours because you do not smoke. There are so many nuances that determine someone's experience after surgery, basing your decision on a few other's experiences may lead you down the wrong path.

I also think that the further out someone is from surgery, the more seriously you should take their advice. Because weight loss success should be measured over the long run, we should listen to the stories of those who are five or more years out from their surgery to get a complete picture. Your relationship with food is very different at five years out from surgery than it is at three.

Perhaps one exception to my caution against basing your decision on the experience of one person is when that person is a first degree, blood relative. If your parent, child or sibling has undergone surgery, then there is a much higher likelihood that your experience will be similar to theirs[98]. Again, genetics is the most important determinant of your outcome after surgery. When you watch a family member go through Bariatric Surgery, we are offered a glimpse of how your DNA will impact your results. As I have mentioned, we don't have any tests that can be used to assess your genetic response to surgery, but the stories of your genetic relatives are the next best things - be sure to take this into consideration if you are lucky enough to have someone you share DNA with go through weight loss surgery.

Today, there are four procedures that are offered in the United States and paid for by most insurance companies. In my opinion, for 99% of all patients, there are only two reasonable options to choose from, the laparoscopic Gastric Bypass and the laparoscopic Sleeve Gastrectomy. These procedures both offer substantial weight loss and a favorable short and long-term safety profile. The other two operations, Adjustable Gastric Banding (like the Lap-Band™) and the Duodenal Switch, in my opinion, have too little reward, and too much risk, respectively.

Before we dig into the nuances of choosing between a Sleeve Gastrectomy and a Gastric Bypass, let's first examine Adjustable Gastric Banding and the Duodenal Switch. If we can gain an understanding of the downsides of these operations, we'll be able to appreciate the upsides of the Sleeve Gastrectomy and Gastric Bypass better.

Adjustable Gastric Banding

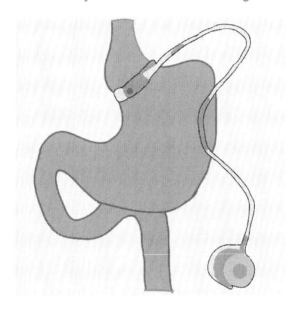

Figure 9 - The Adjustable Gastric Band

The Lap-Band® system was approved by the FDA in 2001 and was touted as a safe alternative to Gastric Bypass[101]. The Lap-Band® was bought and sold by several companies and ultimately came under ownership by Allergan, the multi-billion dollar company behind Botox (the Lap-Band® has recently been sold again to Apollo EndoSurgery). When I started performing Bariatric Surgery in 2006, the Lap-Band® was everywhere. There were commercials on TV, billboards on every highway, giant, two story booths at the Bariatric Surgery meetings and dozens of well-respected experts on Allergan's payroll publishing research and giving talks. The Lap-Band® was presented as the perfect weight loss operation - it reportedly offered patients equivalent weight loss to the Gastric Bypass[102], was easily reversible and had an exceedingly low complication rate[103].

In 2008 and 2009, Adjustable Gastric Banding was the most popular weight loss surgery performed in the United States. Patients not surprisingly flocked to the operation on the promises of weight loss without risk and surgeons paid big bucks to become "certified" to place the bands surgically.

Initially, we all recognized that our Gastric Band patients were losing much less weight than our Gastric Bypass patients, but the research showed that the weight loss was slow and took as long as four to five years until patients lost all their weight. At the height of the Gastric Band craze, we started hearing whispers from many surgeons that the weight loss in their practice did not match the research studies and the long-term complication rate was alarmingly high. Bariatric Surgeons as a group tend to be more extroverted and collaborative than other surgeons. At conferences and meetings, we often share stories of what's working for our patients and what troubles we're having. Over and over, surgeons were sharing their difficulties with Adjustable Gastric Bands. Patients were not losing weight and were having a terrible time with vomiting, difficulty swallowing and heartburn. Despite surgeons following the recommendations from the experts and the device manufacturers, their patients weren't doing as well as they expected.

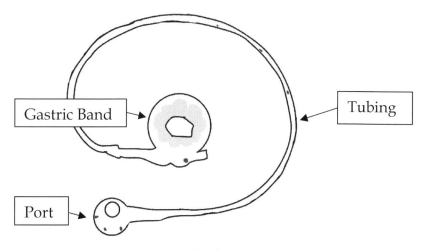

Figure 10 - The Gastric Band - Port, Tubing and Band

Adjustable Gastric Bands have two parts. The main part is an inflatable bladder that wraps around the upper part of the stomach. This part is connected by a tube to the "port," a small, round plastic piece with a rubber center that sits just beneath the patient's skin. Surgeons can inflate the bladder around the stomach by injecting saline via the port that sits underneath the skin. Band adjustment procedures take just a few seconds and can be done in the office. The goal is to slowly inflate the band over a period of a few months until it is just the right tightness. Patients should be able to eat small portions of food and feel satisfied, yet not suffer from frequent vomiting, heartburn or difficulty swallowing.

The primary problem with Adjustable Gastric Bands is that they induce a much smaller hormonal change than other weight loss surgeries[104]. The primary emphasis of the band is to induce restriction - patients can only eat small amounts of food until they feel full. As we have learned, simple calorie restriction alone is bound to fail in the long run, and this is exactly what we were finding in our practice as patients failed to lose weight after their Gastric Band surgery.

In my practice, I've found that most Gastric Band patients fall into one of three groups. The first group is the smallest and represents around 5% of all band patients. This small number of "super-responders" lose weight easily and quickly after surgery, requiring very few band adjustments and naturally decrease their appetite and improve the quality of their diet without much effort. These patients have a very powerful hormonal response to the mere placement of the band, it is rarely necessary to tighten it significantly. For this small group, Adjustable Gastric Bands represent the ideal weight loss surgery. Their results are excellent, the surgical risk is almost negligible and the required follow up care is minimal. Unfortunately, this group represents only a small minority of all the patients who have Adjustable Gastric Bands placed.

The second category of patients are "partial responders" and consist of over half the group. These patients are able to lose between 50-60 pounds easily after surgery. However, after they lose this weight, they plateau and are unable to drop another pound. Again, for reasons we don't fully understand, these patients are able to lower their set point by only 50-60 pounds. Increasing their restriction by injecting more saline into the band does not lower their metabolic thermostat's set point, it just worsens heartburn, difficulty swallowing and vomiting.

The final group of patients lose only a few pounds after surgery, largely because they are placed on a restrictive postoperative diet in the first few months after the procedure. As soon as they resume their normal diet, the weight comes back and they receive no weight loss benefit from the band.

Patients and surgeons alike who try to increase the restriction of the band by inflating it tightly to drive weight loss find themselves trapped on a miserable merry go round. In an effort to achieve additional weight loss, the band is inflated until it is very tight. This enforces calorie restriction, resulting in the usual weight loss we see from calorie restriction alone - 10% of your total body weight. In an effort to achieve even more weight loss, the band is tightened further, usually to the point where the patient has difficulty tolerating solid foods. Because the patient is now living well onto the starvation side of his or her metabolic thermostat, the hunger they experience increases and the patients find themselves seeking out soft, calorie dense foods. These soft foods are able to slide through the super tight band, while healthier foods like fruits and vegetables get stuck.

Living with an extremely tight band is not sustainable and results in a life of frequent vomiting (several times a day), painful swallowing and severe heartburn, particularly at night. Ultimately, these patients return to their surgeon who removes some of the fluid which provides immediate relief. The patient is able to return to their normal diet, which, of course, results in significant weight regain as the patient moves out of the starvation side of their thermostat and back toward their set

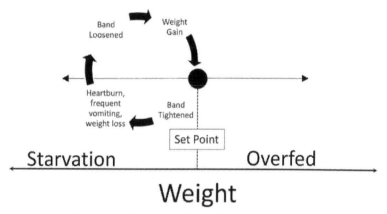

Figure 11- The vicious Gastric Band merry-go-round

point. Frustrated by their weight regain, the patients return back to their surgeon to have the fluid put back in, starting the whole cycle over again.[105,106]

As surgeons across the country recognized that their own clinical experiences were quite different from the marketing research that was presented in the journals and at the conferences, the number of Gastric Band surgeries decreased. The problems of heartburn, difficulty swallowing and frequent vomiting worsen with time. In 2019, very few surgeons continue to offer Adjustable Gastric Bands to their patients and there are more bands removed every year than are placed.[107]

Although very few lap bands are being placed these days, there remain hundreds of thousands of people who still have a band in place. I continue to see these patients frequently in my office and work with them to help them understand what the band can and cannot do for them. Depending on how much weight the patient has lost and what type of symptoms they are having, we can often get patients to a more comfortable place without surgery. In order to follow the Pound of Cure program, the band needs to be relatively loose to allow them to eat the large volumes of vegetables, fruits, nuts, seeds and beans that are required for success. Sometimes we're able to help these patients lose weight, other times, the patient decides to have the band removed and then convert to either a Gastric Bypass or Sleeve Gastrectomy[105]. This is a complicated decision and should be made after careful consideration with a bariatric surgeon who performs revision surgery frequently.

BilioPancreatic Diversion with Duodenal Switch

The BilioPancreatic Diversion with Duodenal Switch (often referred to just as the "Duodenal Switch.") is the most effective weight loss surgery available[108]. It also has the highest rate of complications, and long-term vitamin deficiencies[109]. I do not offer the Duodenal Switch to my patients and refer those who are interested in the surgery to one of the very few surgeons who perform it. Some Duodenal Switch surgeons perform this surgery through a large incision (open), rather than through several small incisions (laparoscopically) as the other bariatric procedures are.

The serious complication rate after Duodenal Switch is 2-3 times higher than after Gastric Bypass[110]. Even more concerning is the remarkably high rate of vitamin deficiencies. Most patients require between $100-$200 per month of vitamin supplements after the procedure that aren't covered by insurance and are critical to maintaining good health[111]. Although the downsides of this surgery are significant, so are the upsides. The Duodenal Switch represents the best treatment for Diabetes and is able to get nearly all diabetic patients off insulin after the surgery[112]. It also offers the most profound weight loss. Most patients are able drop nearly all of their excess weight without making significant changes to their diet. However, nearly every meal results in a trip to the bathroom, particularly if the food has a high fat content[113].

Although some aspects of the surgery seem too good to be true, I have cared for many patients who struggle with the chronic health conditions that their surgically induced malnutrition has created. These patients are often much thinner, but not always much healthier. Their high blood pressure and diabetes are replaced by severe osteoporosis, chronic diarrhea and a general appearance of poor health. While this surgery may be the best option for a small group of patients, particularly those with a very high BMI (>60) or severe diabetes, it should be chosen with great caution and understanding of the risks and nutritional consequences. I believe that a Gastric Bypass or Sleeve Gastrectomy procedure, paired with significant improvement in your diet and exercise program can bring about results that are nearly as good as with the Duodenal Switch, with a fraction of the difficulties.

My practice is almost exactly 50% Sleeve Gastrectomy and 50% Gastric Bypass. I am not a zealot or firm believer that one procedure is superior to the other. They are both excellent operations that are more similar than different in their outcomes and patient experiences. I let my patients make their own choice about which surgery to perform, but always offer my advice on which I think would provide the best results for them.

CHAPTER SEVEN
THE GASTRIC BYPASS

The Gastric Bypass has been performed since the late 1960's[114], and with relative frequency since the 1990's. It is a time-tested procedure that is still performed frequently today. In the 1970's, the patients contemplating bariatric surgery had to choose between the jejunal-ileal bypass and the Gastric Bypass[115]. Few of you have heard of the jejunal-ileal bypass, and for good reason - it's not performed any more. In the 1980's and 1990's, your surgical options included the Gastric Bypass, the vertical banded gastroplasty (commonly referred to as "stomach stapling")[116] and the Bilopancreatic Diversion/ Duodenal Switch[117]. Early this century, the two most frequent surgeries performed were Adjustable Gastric Banding and the Gastric Bypass[118]. Today, most patients decide between the Sleeve Gastrectomy and the Gastric Bypass[119]. This brief history lesson points out that many Bariatric Surgeries have come and gone over the last fifty years, but the Gastric Bypass has always been an option because of its high success rate and low rate of both long- and short-term complications.

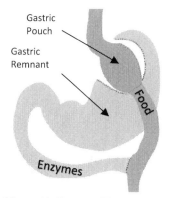

Gastric Pouch

Gastric Remnant

Food

Enzymes

Figure 12- Roux-en-Y Gastric Bypass

The Gastric Bypass (officially the Roux-en-Y Gastric Bypass) operation effectively reroutes your intestines from a straight line into a "Y" shape. Of the two upper limbs of the "Y," one contains the food that you eat while the other houses the digestive enzymes. At the crotch of the "Y," the two limbs come together and the food mixes with the enzymes. This delay in the mixing of food with enzymes (typically this occurs immediately after food leaves the stomach) changes the chemical makeup of the first portion of the intestine. Food bypasses the first portion of the intestine – it only contains acid from the gastric remnant and digestive enzymes. Food also can't enter the large section of bypassed stomach (the gastric remnant) which contains cells that are very active in the release of hunger and satiety hormones. For reasons that we don't fully understand, these changes trick your brain into lowering your metabolic thermostat's set point[53].

Approximately 20% of all the weight loss surgeries performed in 2017 were Gastric Bypass procedures[120]. The Sleeve Gastrectomy has risen in popularity quickly and has become much more popular, however, my recent conversations with other Bariatric Surgeons indicate that the pendulum may be beginning to swing back toward the Gastric Bypass. A Gastric Bypass surgery offers excellent weight loss, minimal weight regain and the serious complication rate runs between 2-3% for most patients[95]. This surgery can be completed through small incisions (laparoscopically) more than 99% of the time[121]. The surgery typically takes between 1-2 hours and requires a hospital stay between 1-3 nights.

The Gastric Bypass is a very powerful set point lowering surgery. It typically results in greater weight loss than the Sleeve Gastrectomy[122,123]. Even more importantly, the Gastric Bypass is probably a more durable operation than the Sleeve Gastrectomy, allowing patients to maintain their weight loss for a longer period of time after surgery[124]. This point is heavily debated, particularly by those surgeons who only perform the Sleeve Gastrectomy and don't feel comfortable performing a Gastric Bypass. Among surgeons (like me) who offer both procedures, there tends to be agreement that Gastric Bypass patients are able to lose more weight and keep it off for a longer period of time.

While most of us look at long term compliance with the recommended postoperative diet as being the sole responsibility of the patient, my personal observations as well as an emerging body of research demonstrate that postoperative compliance is more complicated than we've previously thought[125,126,127].

When we look at Bariatric Surgery as a hormonal, set point lowering procedure, rather than one that works by anatomically restricting your food intake or inducing the malabsorption of nutrients, our perspective on post-operative compliance changes. Because the surgery works by adjusting your hunger and metabolism to drive weight loss, patients who have less hunger after surgery have a much easier time following the postoperative rules. As we've already discussed, the degree of success after surgery varies significantly from individual to individual, as does the amount of hunger that patients have.

Because the Gastric Bypass offers a more powerful hormonal effect than the Sleeve Gastrectomy, patients after Gastric Bypass surgery often have an easier time following our Pound of Cure plan postoperatively[128]. Most patients after Gastric Bypass surgery have a strong preference for fruit, vegetables, nuts, seeds and beans and develop a dislike for greasy or sugary processed foods[54]. Many patients will develop abdominal pain or nausea after eating heavily processed foods. The Gastric Bypass will change your relationship with food and encourage you to not only eat less, but also to choose healthier foods. The simplest way that I explain the difference between the two surgeries is that the Sleeve Gastrectomy will nudge you toward eating a better diet while the Gastric Bypass will shove you toward a healthier diet.

If you are already a healthy eater and prefer nutrient dense foods like those recommended on the Pound of Cure plan, then this added effect of the Gastric Bypass is unnecessary. However, if you have a difficult time making changes to your diet preoperatively, then you should strongly consider the Gastric Bypass since it will offer you the help you need to change your diet after surgery. Some people are attracted to the idea of a surgery that punishes you for eating poorly, while others are not. This is a personal choice that should be considered when you decide which surgery to have.

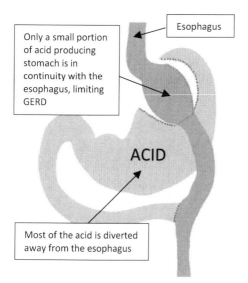

Only a small portion of acid producing stomach is in continuity with the esophagus, limiting GERD

Esophagus

ACID

Most of the acid is diverted away from the esophagus

Figure 13- Gastric Bypass Surgery is an effective treatment of GERD

Many patients who are overweight also suffer from heartburn, also known as GastroEsophageal Reflux Disease or GERD for short. GERD is caused by acid in your stomach travelling back up into your esophagus and irritating the sensitive lining. Gastric Bypass surgery diverts the majority of the acid producing part of the stomach away from the esophagus. The acid just can't get into the esophagus because it's no longer connected. Since GERD is caused by acid irritating the esophageal lining, the Gastric Bypass surgery is a very effective treatment of GERD[129].

Being overweight increases the pressure in your abdomen and this increased pressure pushes the stomach upward, into your chest cavity. When the stomach is pushed up into your chest, this is referred to as a "hiatal hernia." Hiatal hernias are present in 25% -35% of people who are significantly overweight[130,131]. The valve between your esophagus and stomach that prevents GERD doesn't work well if you have a hiatal hernia. Between a poorly functioning valve and increased pressure in your abdominal cavity, obesity is strongly associated with GERD. Hiatal hernias are frequently repaired at the same time as your weight loss surgery, however recurrences are common and repair does not guarantee a lifetime free from heartburn[131]. Because Gastric Bypass surgery is very effective at reducing GERD, it is unnecessary to repair small hiatal hernias, however, larger hiatal hernias should be fixed at the same time[132].

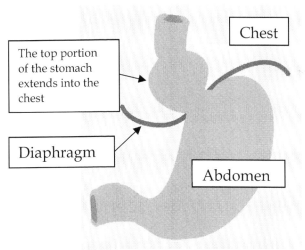

The top portion of the stomach extends into the chest

Chest

Diaphragm

Abdomen

Figure 14- A Hiatal Hernia

There is also a strong dietary component to GERD, and I've found that many people who suffer from GERD are able to find relief just by changing their diet toward a nutrient dense plan[133] like the Pound of Cure. If you continuously suffer from severe GERD despite changing your diet, then you should strongly consider Gastric Bypass Surgery. Gastric Bypass surgery reroutes the majority of the acid in your stomach away from your esophagus, decreasing the severity of GERD significantly. I've found nearly a 100% resolution of GERD symptoms in my practice after Gastric Bypass surgery. The Sleeve Gastrectomy may improve your GERD symptoms, but it can also make it worse[134]. If you suffer from daily symptoms of GERD that are making you miserable, then a Gastric Bypass represents your best surgical option.

I also typically steer patients who suffer from severe Diabetes toward a Gastric Bypass. In the early days of the Gastric Bypass, surgeons quickly realized that the surgery caused patients' diabetes to improve dramatically and even resolve completely, often within a few days of surgery[135]. This finding has completely changed our view of Diabetes from an incurable, chronic disease to one that can be treated and even "cured."[136] If your primary goal of surgery is to resolve your diabetes, then a Gastric Bypass offers your best chance since it is more effective at normalizing your blood sugar than a Sleeve Gastrectomy[137,138].

When deciding on which surgery to undergo, it comes down to performing a thorough investigation of the risks and benefits of each procedure. The benefits of a Gastric Bypass include significant, durable weight loss, a change in your taste preferences toward healthier food and improvement of Diabetes, GERD and many other medical conditions. The recovery is surprisingly fast, and most patients experience only minimal pain and are able to return to work within 2-3 weeks after surgery. However, with all surgeries, there is a risk that things don't go as planned and you suffer a complication after surgery.

I will leave an exhaustive discussion of every possible complication to your surgeon (and the poundofcureweightloss.com website) and will just focus on the problems that are commonly seen or discussed. While things can go terribly wrong after Gastric Bypass surgery, this is very uncommon and is only a serious concern for patients who are at high risk for surgery due to advanced age, a heart condition, severe diabetes or limited mobility. The mortality risk of gastric bypass surgery is lower than gallbladder removal[139]. The risk of serious complications runs between 2-3% for most patients**Error! Bookmark not defined.** and these complications are typically straightforward problems that can be very frightening but are rarely truly life threatening[140]. While most patients' fears of dying on the operating room table or ending up in the Intensive Care Unit for months are understandable, these are extremely uncommon events. When you examine your risks closely, most patients have a decreased risk of death after surgery when the results are averaged over three to five years. While the surgery carries a small risk up front, the benefits of the procedure will decrease your risk of dying from other causes over the long run[141,142].

The primary concern with Gastric Bypass surgery is not what happens within the first month after surgery since these risks are low and the problems are treatable. The primary issue with Gastric Bypass surgery is the problems that can occur years or even decades after surgery. Between 20%-25% of all gastric bypass patients will require another abdominal surgery within the first decade[143,144]. The majority of these abdominal surgeries are gallbladder removal, which is generally safe and well tolerated, but this alarming statistic demonstrates that the excellent weight loss, diabetes resolution and GERD relief offered by a gastric bypass may come at a price.

Iron Deficiency

Many patients are concerned about significant malnutrition and vitamin deficiencies after surgery. While deficiencies that are identified on bloodwork are common, symptoms from these deficiencies are relatively uncommon[145]. Unlike the Duodenal Switch, patients rarely become dependent on extensive vitamin supplements after Gastric Bypass surgery. However, iron deficiency is very common, occurring in up to 25% of all postoperative patients[146]. Iron deficiency after Gastric Bypass surgery is a complicated problem, and its cause remains unclear. The most common explanation is that most iron absorption occurs in the first portion of the small intestine which is bypassed after the surgery. The vast majority of patients who suffer from iron deficiency after surgery respond well to daily oral iron supplements. I treat iron deficient patients with a Bariatric iron formulation that is better tolerated than the most common, non-bariatric iron supplement, Ferrous Sulfate. Ferrous Sulfate is poorly tolerated by most Gastric Bypass patients and causes abdominal cramping and constipation[147]. Bariatric formulations (also known as chelated iron) rarely cause constipation and are equally effective at raising your iron levels.

While most patients respond well to oral iron supplements, around 8% of patients require intravenous iron infusions[148]. Most of the time, these infusions only need to be given over a month or two until the iron levels return to normal. After the infusions, patients can maintain a normal iron level on oral supplements.

For most patients, iron deficiency after surgery is very manageable if you and your doctors stay on top of it. If you ignore your iron levels for several years, you run the risk of developing a severe deficiency that requires regular intravenous infusions and occasionally, a blood transfusion. Most of the time, this could have been prevented if the patient's iron levels were checked and supplements were taken regularly. All Gastric Bypass patients should have their iron level checked yearly, and more frequently if they are low. Daily, appropriate iron supplementation can be a part of life after Gastric Bypass surgery[149].

Internal Hernia/ Intestinal Obstruction

Approximately 2-3% of all Gastric Bypass patients will develop an internal hernia or intestinal obstruction at some point after the surgery[150]. An internal hernia occurs when the intestines become stuck in a twisted position. While this sounds very concerning, this is rarely a life-threatening condition and often is present for months before a diagnosis is made[151]. In a small percentage of cases, internal hernias can be life threatening. Because it's impossible to know which cases are life-threatening, all internal hernias should be fixed promptly, ideally within 24 hours of diagnosis, or sooner if you are in significant pain.

Internal Hernias can be fixed by an experienced bariatric surgeon who can perform the repair laparoscopically. These repairs typically only require a one-night stay in the hospital. Other, non-bariatric surgeons and gastroenterologists often struggle to make this diagnosis and provide safe, minimally invasive treatment because it requires a solid understanding of Gastric Bypass anatomy. Additionally, the primary diagnostic test, a CT scan is often misread by radiologists who aren't familiar with the often subtle findings[152]. For this reason, it is critical that you see a bariatric surgeon if you have significant abdominal pain, even if you are many years out from your surgery. A small fraction of internal hernias or intestinal obstructions cannot be treated laparoscopically and require a traditional, open surgery to repair. These patients have a much longer recovery and often take three full months until they are back to normal.

Ulcers

Ulcers after Gastric Bypass surgery occur most frequently in patients who continue to smoke after surgery. They can occur in non-smokers as well, but less commonly. Gastric Bypass patients who continue to smoke after surgery are at very high risk for the development of ulcers. Also, if you continue to smoke after developing an ulcer, all treatments of the ulcer will fail.

Eventually, the ulcer will either begin to bleed or perforate, requiring an emergent surgery[153].

Ulcers typically cause pain very high up in your abdomen, just underneath your breastbone, particularly with eating. They also cause a significant decrease in your appetite. Patients with significant ulcers will often start to lose weight again several years after surgery. I can often diagnose ulcers in the office within a few seconds of meeting the patient. The smell of tobacco on the patient is my first clue, but what confirms the diagnosis is the sunken face, pale, almost grey colored skin and a general appearance of poor health. Occasionally, patients tell me that they do not want to have a Gastric Bypass performed because they have a friend who had the surgery and now looks terrible. When I ask if this person smokes, the answer is almost always yes.

A second cause of ulcers after Gastric Bypass is the regular use of non-steroidal anti-inflammatory medications (NSAIDs) like Ibuprofen, Naproxen or Aspirin. This is the reason that Gastric Bypass patients are instructed to avoid these medications. While taking NSAIDs a few times a month poses very little risk, regular use can put you at significant risk.

When ulcers occur in non-smoking patients, they are easier to treat than in smokers. Even if you quit smoking immediately after being diagnosed with an ulcer, the effects of smoking will linger for months and delaying healing. If you are a non-smoker, a one to two-month course of treatment with aggressive antacids allows the ulcer to heal, however, between 5%-10% of the time, surgery is needed to treat the ulcer[154]. I've found that surgery is very effective in treating ulcers that are resistant to medications if the patient quits smoking first, or never smoked in the first place. Patients that continue to smoke after ulcer surgery are likely to develop another ulcer within a year or two.

Hair loss

Most Gastric Bypass patients experience some hair loss after surgery. For some, it's just a few more hairs on the brush, while others report that it comes out in clumps. It typically starts around three to five months after surgery and is at its worst between months six and nine. However, after the first year, your hair begins to grow back and is typically back to normal around two years after surgery. The longer your hair is, the longer it will take before it returns to normal. Also, those who start with thick hair typically have less problems than those with thin or fine hair to begin with.

The exact cause of the hair loss is unclear, however most of us suspect that it is the result of rapid weight loss and poor nutrition during the first few months after surgery. While I typically push a "vegetables first" approach to postoperative eating, I suspend this for up to a year after surgery to ensure that patients in the immediate postoperative period get adequate protein intake. During these first few months after surgery, I encourage patients to "eat their protein first" to minimize hair loss.

The most common nutritional cause of hair loss is iron deficiency. If I see hair loss in a patient more than one year out from surgery, their iron level is almost always low when I check it. While I don't start most patients out on iron, if you have a history of anemia or want to do everything possible to minimize hair loss, then taking a bariatric specific, chelated iron supplement starting immediately after Gastric Bypass surgery is a reasonable approach. Also, starting a high dose biotin supplement (10,000 micrograms daily) immediately after surgery may also minimize hair loss. While zinc has often been cited as a cause of hair loss, I do not recommend patients empirically take zinc supplements since it can interfere with iron absorption and may actually worsen your hair loss by predisposing you to iron deficiency. While hair loss is a very troublesome side effect, it is almost always temporary and can be minimized by taking a proactive approach of increased protein intake and daily biotin and iron supplementation.

Gas

Copious, foul smelling gas can occur after Gastric Bypass in some patients. While excessive gas is typically a topic for humor, I have a few patients who will tell me that it's nothing to laugh about. We now understand that the Gastric Bypass works to lower your body's weight set point, but the mechanism that drives this is largely unknown. One popular theory is that the surgical rearrangement of the intestines changes the type of bacteria present within the GI tract. As we learn more about the different bacteria that live in our intestines, we are discovering that they impact our body's function in many different ways. There is research that suggests that the bacteria in our intestines are responsible for the increased rates of autism[155], multiple sclerosis[156], Crohn's disease[157] and obesity[158].

It is possible that the change in the bacteria population that favorably impacts our weight may also result in excessive gas. There is hope for those who suffer from excessive, foul smelling gas after a Gastric Bypass. A very inexpensive, over the counter medication called Devrom can be very helpful, as can taking Beano (also over the counter) before eating beans and vegetables. Probiotics and digestive enzymes can also be helpful in decreasing excessive gas[159]. Most patients do not notice a significant change in the amount or smell of their gas, however it can be a distressing side effect for the few that do.

Gallstones

Gallstones are very common in the United States but occur even more frequently after weight loss surgery. The most common explanation for the increased rate after a Gastric Bypass is that rapid weight loss triggers a change in the makeup of your bile that causes the stones to form in your gallbladder[160]. Your gallbladder is an organ that stores bile that we use in digestion and likely played a much bigger role in the digestion of our caveman ancestors than it does today. As I've pointed out many times, our body's physiology evolved in response to our prehistoric environment and is not particularly well suited for today's modern environment. It's likely that the gallbladder evolved to aid in digesting the large amount of meat and animal fat that cavemen would consume after a successful hunt. Most cavemen ate meat at most a few times per week[161], and when they did, it was very large portions because the meat rotted very quickly. The gallbladder allows for a large amount of bile to be released at one time which would likely be useful for a caveman indulging after a big hunt.

Today's modern diet typically does not consist of several pounds of raw or poorly cooked meat in a single sitting, so the gallbladder is no longer as important for digestion. When stones develop in the gallbladder, patients typically experience pain in the upper abdomen or on their right side, particularly after eating a fatty meal. Even foods like nuts and avocados can trigger the pain. An ultrasound examination of the abdomen can successfully make, or rule out the presence of gallstones, 99% of the time[162]. Successful treatment of gallstones requires that the entire gallbladder is removed. Any attempts to dissolve the stones through diet or sonic waves are ineffective, and even if they do help, the stones will re-form within weeks. A cholecystectomy, or removal of the gallbladder, can be performed as an outpatient procedure most of the time and typically requires just a few days off work. The risks of suffering a complication after gallbladder removal is relatively low, however, if you are a post-gastric bypass patient, your risk of developing a complication after gallbladder removal is almost twice as high as normal[163].

Gallstones do pose a particular risk to Gastric Bypass patients because of the changes in anatomy that are made during the surgery. Gallstones can travel out of the gallbladder and into the main liver duct where they can get stuck. When this happens in a patient who has not had Gastric Bypass surgery, we can place an endoscope through your mouth, and into your intestines to retrieve the gallstones through the scope. While these patients still need to have their gallbladder removed, they avoid a major surgery to retrieve the stones directly from the main liver duct.

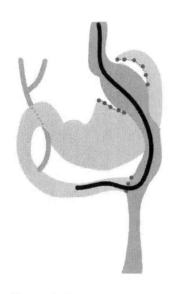

Figure 15 - ERCP is difficult after Gastric Bypass

After a Gastric Bypass, it is no longer a simple matter of removing the stones by performing an endoscopy through your mouth since the main part of your stomach is separated during the surgery. In my practice, I've managed to avoid the need for a major surgery by going to the operating room, removing the gallbladder and making a small hole in the old stomach and having the endoscopist remove the stones through the hole in the stomach[164]. While this requires a little longer recovery than a straightforward removal of the gallbladder, it is still not nearly as risky or difficult as when the stones are surgically removed directly from the main liver duct. Sleeve Gastrectomy patients are also prone to the development of gallstones after surgery, however because they do not have any disruption in the arrangement of their intestines, they can still undergo an endoscopic removal of gallstones if they get stuck in the main liver duct.

For this reason, I recommend that patients who have had a Gastric Bypass undergo a gallbladder removal if they ever develop gallstones, rather than taking a "wait and see" approach. If you are in the process of working toward Gastric

Bypass surgery and have gallstones that are causing symptoms, I recommend having your gallbladder removed at the same time as the Gastric Bypass procedure, or even a few months before to prevent this problem. In the early days of Gastric Bypass surgery, the gallbladder was removed routinely, however this practice is no longer advised since it results in the unnecessary removal of many normal gallbladders[165].

Alcoholism

The final issue that I talk to prospective Gastric Bypass patients about is the development of Alcoholism after surgery. For a long time, most of us described the increased rate of alcoholism after Gastric Bypass surgery as the result of a "transfer addiction." The belief was that because weight loss surgery minimized a person's ability to indulge their food addiction, they sought out other substances, like alcohol. However, as our understanding of these surgeries evolved, we began to recognize that the transfer addiction model did not fully explain the increased rate of alcoholism. First, we determined that the rate of addiction to alcohol after surgery was much higher than to other drugs or tobacco[166]. Second, post-operative patients were reporting that their body's response to alcohol changed after surgery[167]. Finally, we were seeing a much higher rate of addiction after Gastric Bypass, compared to other Bariatric procedures[168].

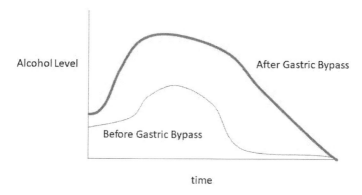

Alcohol Level

After Gastric Bypass

Before Gastric Bypass

time

Figure 16 - Alcohol is absorbed differently after Gastric Bypass surgery

Patients after both procedures reported that they became more intoxicated after drinking less alcohol than they did before surgery. They also reported that the intoxication lasted longer. When we examined alcohol levels in postoperative patients, we found that their absorption pattern differed from those who have not had surgery. We found that alcohol levels increased faster, went higher and stayed high for longer, supporting the patients' reports[167].

These results were profound in some patients, while others experienced less sensitivity. In many patients, a single alcoholic beverage caused them to develop blood alcohol levels over the legal limit for driving[169].

It's very difficult to determine the exact rate of the development of new alcohol problems after surgery, however, our best estimate is that around 3% of all Gastric Bypass patients will develop a new alcohol use problem after surgery[170]. This is a very important statistic for anyone considering Gastric Bypass surgery to take seriously. The change in your alcohol absorption pattern will change your relationship with alcohol. Many patients report that they no longer enjoy alcohol at all and have found that their consumption decreases. However, for some, this new absorption pattern triggers pleasure centers in the brain that weren't stimulated by alcohol before surgery. These patients now have the potential to develop an alcohol problem if they continue to drink. If you notice that you enjoy alcohol much more after surgery than you did before, it is absolutely critical that you stop drinking completely before the problem escalates. You are choosing to undergo Bariatric Surgery in order to make your life better. After more than a decade of performing these surgeries, I have a handful of patients who now struggle with alcoholism. I can assure you that, although the surgery has made these patients thinner, their life is not better.

From 2010 to 2017, the pendulum swung away from Gastric Bypass toward the Sleeve Gastrectomy due to the public's perception that the Sleeve Gastrectomy offered similar weight loss results without as much risk. While there is certainly merit to the argument that the complication rate is lower, our long-term experience with the Sleeve is bringing our belief that both procedures offer similar weight loss into question. We are now starting to see the pendulum swing slowly back toward the Gastric Bypass. As you will see in our next section, both procedures have strengths and weaknesses. For some patients, the decision between a Gastric Bypass and Sleeve Gastrectomy is straightforward, but for most, it is very difficult. If you are struggling to choose the best operation for you, then you are probably doing a good job in considering all of the important factors. It's likely that there is not one best choice, but two very good options that offer different benefits and risks. In the end, a thoughtful, open conversation with a bariatric surgeon who performs both surgeries should help you to decide.

CHAPTER EIGHT
SLEEVE GASTRECTOMY

The Sleeve Gastrectomy has only been performed as a primary weight loss procedure for a little more than ten years[171]. The Sleeve started to become popular around the same time that we were beginning to recognize the shortcomings of Adjustable Gastric Banding. Its popularity increased rapidly and since 2015 has been the most commonly performed weight loss procedure in the United States[120].

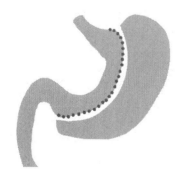

Figure 17- A Sleeve Gastrectomy is performed by removing approximately 80% of your stomach

The Sleeve is a more straightforward procedure that transforms the stomach into a narrow tube, shaped very much like a shirt sleeve by removing around 80% of the stomach. Some people think that we place a "sleeve" around the stomach and that, down the road, the sleeve can be removed if necessary, however, there are no foreign bodies placed during Gastric Sleeve surgery. **The "Sleeve" is fashioned by removing a portion of the stomach and this is not at all reversible.**

While most people look at the Sleeve as a surgery that works primarily by reducing your ability to eat large portions, the Sleeve exerts its primary weight loss effect through hormonal changes, just like the Gastric Bypass[172]. The portion of the stomach that is removed plays a critical role in your metabolic thermostat's inner workings and removing it causes an immediate lowering of your set point.

Because the stomach is removed completely, this surgery is completely irreversible, in contrast to a Gastric Bypass that can be reversed, but at high risk. Many patients have downplayed the Sleeve as a minor surgery, but the removal of 80% of your stomach should not be taken lightly. I often pose the following question to Sleeve Gastrectomy patients that I think are taking their decision too lightly: "If you were checking in to the hospital tomorrow to have 80% of your stomach removed, would you consider it a minor surgery?" Even though a Sleeve Gastrectomy can be performed extremely safely with only a 1-2% serious complication rate[95], it is not a minor surgery.

Many centers have embraced the novelty of the Sleeve and have moved toward this surgery exclusively, no longer performing Gastric Bypass surgery. This trend has started to reverse and the Sleeve zealots who have abandoned all other Bariatric procedures are decreasing in number.

The Sleeve Gastrectomy sits immediately between Adjustable Gastric Banding and the Gastric Bypass in both its risk profile and weight loss effect[123]. Compared to Adjustable Gastric Banding, it is a better surgery that offers more weight loss; however, the complication rate of the Sleeve is higher within the first 30 days of surgery. Also, it carries the risk of a leak which is a very rare, but devastating complication.

Compared to the Gastric Bypass, the Sleeve is a safer operation that requires a shorter recovery time, but the Sleeve offers less weight loss than the Gastric Bypass. Not only do patients lose fewer pounds after a Sleeve Gastrectomy, but the weight loss is less durable with a higher rate of weight regain after a few years[122]. Because the Sleeve only involves the stomach, the hormonal changes that lower your metabolic thermostat's set point are less powerful than the Gastric Bypass that offers both stomach and intestinal effects[173]. The result is less weight loss and a less durable result.

Additionally, for those who are severely overweight, a Sleeve Gastrectomy may not represent your best option. If you calculate your BMI (body mass index – determined by taking your weight in kilograms and dividing it by your height in meters squared – use an online calculator, it's much simpler) and it is greater than 50, then you'll lose a lot less weight if you choose to undergo a Sleeve Gastrectomy instead of a Gastric Bypass[174].

Taste Changes

Because the hormonal, set point lowering effects of the Sleeve are less powerful than the Gastric Bypass, there are differences in your taste changes after surgery. While both procedures initially offer significant changes in food preferences and appetite, theses changes lasted longer in Gastric Bypass patients[175]. Gastric Bypass patients are more likely to develop sustained preferences for more natural, unprocessed foods and remained uninterested in processed foods for years after surgery. Sleeve Gastrectomy patients tend to tolerate and occasionally even enjoy processed foods within a few months of surgery. This is a general observation and there is significant variation from person to person. I have certainly seen profound and powerful, sustained taste changes in some Sleeve Gastrectomy patients.

I believe that patients with a healthier starting diet tend to be better candidates for the Sleeve Gastrectomy. Because the Sleeve is less likely to help you develop a sustained change in the types of foods that you prefer, those patients who already enjoy the healthy, unprocessed foods that make up the Pound of Cure program will find this program easy to follow postoperatively. Those patients who struggle to eliminate processed, sweetened foods from their diet preoperatively need more help in order to make the necessary lifestyle changes after surgery. If you are struggling in your efforts to adopt the Pound of Cure eating style before surgery, I believe that you may benefit more from a Gastric Bypass since it will offer you more assistance in changing your food preferences.

While the better safety profile of a Sleeve Gastrectomy and the ability to maintain a more natural straight-line intestinal anatomy (compared to a "Y" shape after Gastric Bypass) is desirable, it's important to recognize that these advantages come at a cost. The Sleeve Gastrectomy is a less effective weight loss surgery when compared to a Gastric Bypass. This does not mean that you are making a mistake by choosing a Sleeve Gastrectomy, it just means that you are choosing to compromise your weight loss results for increased safety and more natural gastrointestinal anatomy.

Heartburn/ GERD

While a Sleeve Gastrectomy is an excellent weight loss surgery with a very low complication rate, heartburn and GERD symptoms after surgery are a significant issue that cannot be ignored. As discussed in the last chapter, patients who have significant heartburn or GERD should strongly consider a Gastric Bypass, rather than a Sleeve Gastrectomy. While most of us experience some heartburn from time to time, there is a small group of patients who experience significant, daily heartburn that often interferes with sleep or their ability to enjoy a meal with friends. If heartburn is a daily part of your life, then a Gastric Bypass will most likely eliminate these symptoms[176], while the heartburn reducing effects of a Sleeve Gastrectomy are more variable. Some patients experience improvement of their heartburn symptoms after a Sleeve Gastrectomy, many stay the same and others report worse symptoms after surgery[177].

A significant percentage of patients will experience worsening of their heartburn and GERD symptoms after surgery[178,179]. These patients may develop occasional or even frequent vomiting after eating as well. The cause of this is believed to be a narrowing or kinking of the mid-portion of the stomach or a breakdown in the anatomy of the valve that sits between your esophagus and stomach that helps to prevent acid from refluxing up into your esophagus. This partial obstruction from the narrowing or kinking increases the pressure in your stomach, and the increased pressure, along with a malfunctioning valve can result in significant acid reflux and heartburn.

For many post-surgical complications, there is relatively little difference between experienced surgeons. However, when it comes to GERD and heartburn symptoms after Sleeve Gastrectomy, there is a significant difference between surgeons. The incidence between surgeons can range from 18% to 45% - a 2 ½ times difference[180]. This difference was not dependent on the age, experience or complication rate of the surgeon. In fact, we really have very little idea of what accounts for this significant difference.

Unfortunately, heartburn rates after surgery are not made public and it can be very difficult to determine if your surgeon has a low rate of postoperative GERD. Perhaps the best way to get more information is to ask your surgeon how often his patients require heartburn medications after surgery. If he or she downplays the significance of heartburn after Sleeve Gastrectomy, they are likely not acknowledging this significant postoperative issue. If they recognize that heartburn does occur after Sleeve Gastrectomy and have a strategy for reducing it, it's likely their patients have a low rate of GERD after surgery.

While many patients will experience heartburn after a Sleeve Gastrectomy, there's a significant percentage (7% - 9%)[179, 181] who suffer symptoms that are so severe that they choose to undergo revision to a Gastric Bypass. The good news for these patients is that revision to a Gastric Bypass is an incredibly effective treatment for their heartburn and GERD[182], but the bad news is that they were essentially forced to have a Gastric Bypass – a surgery they specifically decided against when they first chose to move forward with weight loss surgery.

Many patients learn to live with their heartburn symptoms and do not seek treatment beyond heartburn medications. If you choose not to seek further treatment for severe GERD and heartburn, you increase your risk of developing a condition known as Barrett's esophagus[183]. Barrett's esophagus occurs when the lining of the esophagus changes from normal esophageal cells to those that resemble intestinal or stomach cells in response to constant exposure to refluxed acid. This change unfortunately increases your risk of developing esophageal cancer in the future by 10x or more[184].

Treatment of severe GERD after a Sleeve Gastrectomy can be very challenging. Some patients will respond to high doses of GERD medications like Prilosec® or Prevacid®. For those that don't, there are several options beyond revision to a Gastric Bypass, however these should be considered experimental without any evidence that demonstrates that they are an equally effective treatment. Some options are to endoscopically apply radiofrequency waves to the lower esophagus[185], to surgically remove the narrowed segment and then reconnect it[186] and even to place a magnetic device around the esophagus to block the acid reflux[187]. All of these strategies have marginal success rates. Often times, patients with severe GERD after a Sleeve also have a hiatal hernia where the top part of the Sleeve pushes up into the chest. While repairing this hiatal hernia can be effective, its long-term success rate is relatively low (~50%)[188].

Without question, the most effective treatment for severe GERD or frequent vomiting after a Sleeve Gastrectomy is to convert the Sleeve to a Gastric Bypass. This treatment is nearly 100% effective[182], however, it results in a patient ending up with the long-term consequences of Gastric Bypass surgery after initially choosing a Sleeve Gastrectomy. All patients who elect to undergo a Sleeve Gastrectomy must understand that a small, but not insignificant number of Sleeve Gastrectomy patients may ultimately need to undergo revision to a Gastric Bypass.

Gallstones

Gallstones are a frequent problem that occur 8% of the time after all weight loss surgery[160]. There is no significant difference between the rate of gallstone formation after Sleeve Gastrectomy or Gastric Bypass. Gallstones are typically caused by rapid weight loss, rather than an alteration in your liver function. Some surgeons will prescribe Actigall®, a medication that helps to thin the bile in an effort to prevent the formation of gallstones. While this medication can prevent the formation of gallstones in the first six months after surgery, it has minimal effect over the long run[189].

In the early days of weight loss surgery, surgeons would routinely remove patients' gallbladders at the same time as their surgery. Before 2005, most weight loss surgery was done through a large incision in the abdomen which resulted in the formation of significant scar tissue that made subsequent removal of the gallbladder more difficult. Today, 99% of all weight loss surgeries are performed laparoscopically through 5-7 small incisions which result in very little scar formation making removal of the gallbladder no more difficult than it is in those who have never had any abdominal surgery at all. Since more than 90% of all weight loss surgery patients do not develop gallstones, routine removal of the gallbladder is no longer recommended[190].

Nonetheless, any patient who develops abdominal pain or nausea after eating should consult with their bariatric surgeon to ensure that they have not developed gallstones. A simple ultrasound test will determine the presence of gallstones with 99% accuracy[191] and gallbladder removal can usually be done on an outpatient basis.

Leak

A leak in the staple line after a Sleeve Gastrectomy is without question, the most devastating surgical complication in all of weight loss surgery. A leak allows for the bacteria to escape from the intestinal tract into the abdominal cavity resulting in a dangerous infection that results in sepsis. While leaks can occur after Gastric Bypass as well, they are slightly more frequent after a Sleeve Gastrectomy and are much more difficult to treat. Thankfully, leaks after either procedure occur in less than 1% of patients[192].

A leak after a Sleeve Gastrectomy is usually the result of a Sleeve that is too tight that causes the pressure inside the Sleeve to build up and ultimately burst the staple line, typically at the very top of the Sleeve where the stomach is the thinnest and the pressure is the highest[193]. Because the pressure is high inside the Sleeve, repairing a leak is not a simple matter of suturing the hole closed since it will just reopen again[194]. The analogy that I use with my patients is that repairing a leak after a Sleeve is like trying to seal a connection between two garden hoses when someone is kinking the hose downstream. No matter how well you seal the connection, the downstream blockage increases the water pressure forcing the water to leak out through even the tiniest pinhole.

While leaks after Gastric Bypass have a very high survival rate and can often be completely resolved within a few weeks, leaks after a Sleeve Gastrectomy require much longer treatment in the hospital with the need for multiple subsequent procedures and have a 10% mortality risk[195]. Thankfully, leaks after a Sleeve Gastrectomy occur infrequently and have decreased significantly over the last few years as surgeons have learned the pitfalls of making the Sleeve too tight, particularly at the midportion of the stomach.

Every patient who undergoes weight loss surgery understands that the risk of complications is very low, but not zero. While leaks and other severe complications can and do occur, they are very rare events. The complication rate of weight loss surgery is very similar to other procedures like appendectomy and gallbladder removal[196]. While we understand that all surgery presents a risk of complications, problems after weight loss surgery are typically judged more harshly than after other procedures. This is likely because the public continues to look at weight loss surgery as "taking the easy way out," rather than as a procedure that extends lives, cures disease and dramatically improves the quality of life of the patient. For every devastating weight loss surgery complication, there are dozens and dozens of patients who never experience heart attacks, kidney failure, strokes and even cancers that result from untreated obesity. Study after study demonstrates that the health benefits of weight loss surgery strongly outweigh the risk of post-operative complications[197,198,199].

I discuss the potential for complications with every prospective weight loss surgery patient from the very beginning of the process but find very few in whom the risk of surgery outweighs the potential benefits. If you become consumed with fear over the risk of complications, make sure you also consider the problems that can occur if you don't turn your health around and take the critical steps necessary to control your weight and your future health. Statistically, your risk of suffering a complication from diabetes, heart and lung disease or even developing an obesity related cancer of the breast, prostate, colon or ovary far outweighs the risk of having a surgical complication.

Weight Regain

Without question, my greatest concern for any patient who has undergone a Sleeve Gastrectomy is weight regain after surgery. While it is certainly possible after a Gastric Bypass, it happens more often after a Sleeve Gastrectomy[200].

Most people look at weight regain after surgery as the result of a patient returning to his or her old habits. While a failure to adopt a new, healthier nutritional and exercise plan after surgery will certainly increase your risks of weight regain, there are other factors that are equally important[201]. Just as we've come to recognize that weight gain and obesity are unfair discriminators, we find that weight regain after bariatric surgery follows a similar pattern. In my practice, I've found that some patients have a very strong hormonal response to a Sleeve Gastrectomy and easily maintain their weight loss, while others are very compliant with our high nutrient Pound of Cure program and still manage to regain a few pounds every year. Just as weight gain is not always an accurate indicator of someone's diet, weight regain also may be caused by other factors beyond what a patient eats.

My experience and an increasing number of studies show that the Sleeve Gastrectomy offers less of a hormonal response after surgery that results in a less tightly anchored set point, compared to a Gastric Bypass[128]. Many patients view the Sleeve Gastrectomy as a procedure that offers lifelong restriction, weight loss and long-term weight maintenance by permanently limiting your ability to eat large servings of food. While a Sleeve Gastrectomy initially offers patients excellent portion control, over time, this effect wanes. As they get further out from surgery, Sleeve patients are able to eat larger volumes of food and feel less in control of their appetite and ability to maintain their lost weight[202].

Shortly after surgery, Sleeve Gastrectomy patients are able to eat only a few bites of food and satisfy their appetite. In the immediate months after surgery, patients typically eat fewer than 800 calories daily[203]. When this low-calorie diet is paired with the set point lowering effect of the surgery, most patients are able to easily lose a significant amount of weight. As time passes and the patient's body weight approaches their new, lowered set point weight, their hunger and appetite return. A failure to understand this long-term change can lead patients into a dangerous pattern of thinking that I refer to as the "Portion Control Trap."

The Portion Control Trap can be best explained by examining a postoperative patient's relationship with one of America's favorite foods, pizza. Around six months after surgery, some patients will report to me that they will eat pizza once or twice a week, but it's only a few bites, so what's the harm? When we look forward, we find that this behavior can put a patient on track to regain weight. At six months, they can only eat a few bites, but if we fast forward to a year after surgery, we will find that the same patient now requires one small piece of pizza in order to satisfy his appetite. At two years out from surgery, it is now two small pieces, and at five years out from surgery, we will find the same patient consuming 2-3 normal sized pieces of pizza twice a week.

Weight regain after surgery is an insidious disease that is often driven by a slow and gradual return to your pre-operative eating habits[204]. A solid postoperative nutritional plan focuses on the quality of food, rather than the quantity[205]. The processed foods that fill the aisles of our grocery stores and are served up daily in most restaurants are largely responsible for our country's obesity epidemic and are a threat to the postoperative patient's ability to maintain the precious hormonal changes and weight loss that the surgery has provided. Rationalizing a return to eating these foods postoperatively on a regular basis by explaining that you are only eating a few bites represent the first steps on the path to weight regain. The Portion Control Trap is a threat to all postoperative patients, but particularly Sleeve Gastrectomy patients.

A patient who undergoes a Gastric Bypass will often experience abdominal pain, bloating and diarrhea after eating processed foods, while Sleeve Gastrectomy patients rarely suffer these negative consequences[206]. Both Sleeve and Bypass patients will experience an increase in appetite in the years following surgery, but the Sleeve patient is particularly subject to the Portion Control Trap because their return to eating processed foods will be better tolerated. If your preoperative diet does not include significant amounts of processed foods, then the Sleeve Gastrectomy represents an excellent choice since you are at low risk for falling into the Portion Control Trap. However, if you are looking at a Sleeve Gastrectomy simply as a tool that will prevent or block you from eating too much for the rest of your life, you should closely re-examine your procedure choice.

Many patients spend a considerable amount of time worrying about choosing the correct procedure. While one procedure may represent an ideal choice, it is rare that this decision alone will determine whether you meet your goals after surgery. In the end, success after surgery is determined by your commitment to a healthier lifestyle and your ability to make good choices about food and exercise every day.

CHAPTER NINE
REVISIONS

Revisional Surgery is a complicated topic that requires special consideration. Revision Bariatric Surgery refers to any procedures that are performed after the initial weight loss surgery. They are more complicated surgeries that typically carry higher risk and offer less reward. In some situations, they offer patients a second chance at weight loss and can be lifesaving. Other times, they are overly risky and offer little advantage.

Revisions depend on the initial surgery. A patient who has had a Gastric Bypass procedure has completely different revision options compared to a patient who underwent a Gastric Band procedure. The initial surgery results in the formation of scar tissue which makes the revision surgery more difficult and the surgeon can only modify existing anatomy which often limits the available surgical options.

Those patients who are looking to revise their Gastric Band procedure to another surgery present the greatest opportunity for success after revision. Removal of the Gastric Band and conversion to either a Sleeve Gastrectomy or Gastric Bypass is the most common revisional procedure performed in the United States[207]. These procedures can be offered with a similar safety profile to initial bariatric operations. I typically counsel my revision patients that removing a Gastric Band adds 1% to the serious complication rate, allowing revision to a Sleeve to have only a 2%-3% serious complication rate and revision to a Gastric Bypass presents a 3%-4% risk of serious complication[208].

The decision to convert a Gastric Band to either a Sleeve Gastrectomy or a Gastric Bypass is often difficult. First, many patients who have a Gastric Band in place suffer from significant heartburn symptoms which will improve dramatically or even resolve after revision to a Gastric Bypass but may persist after revision to a Sleeve. However, the heartburn symptoms are likely the result of the band and will often clear up after either procedure, as long as the band is removed. For this reason, GERD is often less of a deciding factor in procedure choice when considering Gastric Band revisions. Second, most patients who undergo revision are doing so because of weight regain or failure to lose enough weight. A Gastric Bypass offers better weight loss[209] and a lower chance of weight regain, however, most patients who initially underwent a Gastric Band chose it over a Gastric Bypass for a specific reason that may still be pertinent today.

When calculating the amount of weight that you can expect to lose after a revisional surgery, a critical piece of information is whether you've lost weight from your Gastric Band procedure. If you've managed to lose and maintain 50 lbs. since your Gastric Band and are choosing to undergo a revision to lose additional weight, you typically lose 50 lbs. less than someone who is having the same procedure for the first time. This makes sense when you consider that all weight loss procedures, even the Gastric Band work by lowering your set point. When you perform a band to bypass revision, you are removing the band which lowered your set point by 50 lbs and then performing a Gastric Bypass which may lower your set point by 125 lbs. Your weight loss from your band to bypass revision will only be 75 lbs., not 125 lbs.[210]

If you've had a Gastric Bypass procedure and have had weight regain, you have very limited options for revision. There are several procedures that are offered, but few of them are particularly effective. The most common revision of a Gastric Bypass is to move the lower connection point further down the intestinal tract, causing more malabsorption. This can result in some weight loss, but usually not the amount desired. Most patients who undergo this procedure lose between 30-60 lbs. but have an increased rate of vitamin and iron deficiencies, and occasionally, significant diarrhea[211]. There are some surgeons who offer a pouch reduction surgery. This procedure trims the gastric pouch and requires that the connection between the stomach and the intestine is redone. This offers a similar amount of weight loss to the malabsorptive revision but does not cause the same iron and vitamin deficiencies. Both of these revisions can be performed laparoscopically, carry a serious complication rate around 5%-10% and usually result in a more difficult recovery than the initial Gastric Bypass[212].

Over the years, there have been multiple endoscopic procedures that have been performed to tighten the opening between the stomach and the intestine. In these procedures, a scope is place through the patient's mouth and either a suturing device or scarring agent is applied to close down the opening between the stomach and the intestine, reducing the patient's ability to eat large portions. These procedures are much safer than the surgical revisions, but typically offer less weight loss and almost all patients experience weight regain within a year[213].

When I see patients in my office with weight regain after a Gastric Bypass, I rarely discuss surgical options and instead work to get patients on our Pound of Cure diet. If exercise is possible, I work to get the patient moving as much as possible. Once we optimize nutrition and exercise, I often add weight loss medications. With these techniques, I can usually help these patients lose 20-40 lbs. without the risk of a revisional surgery.

While Sleeve Gastrectomy patients have a higher rate of weight regain, they have more surgical options to treat weight regain. The most straightforward revision for patients who have regained weight after Sleeve Gastrectomy is to perform a Gastric Bypass. While this is straightforward and is an excellent treatment for post-Sleeve Gastrectomy heartburn symptoms, it is not particularly effective in driving significant weight loss. The weight loss from this revision procedure is typically between 30 to 50 lbs.[214]

Patients who have regained weight after a Sleeve can undergo an intestinal bypass, effectively converting their Sleeve Gastrectomy into a Duodenal Switch. While this revision can offer between 50-80 lbs. of additional weight loss, it is also accompanied by the long-term side effects of the Duodenal Switch procedure. The intestinal diversion that is added to convert a Sleeve Gastrectomy to a Duodenal Switch results in significant vitamin deficiencies, malnutrition and diarrhea[215].

A new procedure, the Single Anastomosis Duodenal-Ileal Bypass (often referred to as the SADI bypass) offers similar weight loss to a Duodenal Switch with fewer side effects. This procedure remains in the experimental phase and is performed by relatively few surgeons in the U.S. Our national society for Bariatric Surgery recommends that this procedure should be limited to experimental protocols and studied more extensively before it is widely offered[216].

A SADI bypass may soon become the best treatment for weight regain after a Sleeve Gastrectomy. It typically results in 50-100 lbs. of weight loss with less of the diarrhea, iron and vitamin deficiencies that are seen with revision to a Duodenal Switch. It is too soon to know whether this weight loss is durable, however the SADI bypass's similarity to the Duodenal Switch would suggest that these patients will be able to maintain their weight loss for many years. The early reports of this procedure report excellent safety with complications rates consistent with the low numbers that we're seeing for primary Gastric Bypass and Sleeve Gastrectomy procedures[217]. Despite the promise of the SADI bypass, patients who opt to have a Sleeve Gastrectomy, rather than a Gastric Bypass may find themselves years later faced with the decision to undergo a second procedure for weight loss that has more long-term side effects than a Gastric Bypass.

Many people point to weight regain in the years following a Bariatric procedure as proof that the surgery does not address the underlying lifestyle issues that cause obesity. However, this viewpoint is overly simplistic and does not properly recognize obesity for what it is, a chronic disease. Obesity is a genetic, physiologic, environmental, social and behavioral disease that is very complex and poorly understood. Surgery currently represents our best treatment for obesity and offers patients a reasonably safe alternative to spending their life trapped underneath a hundred or more pounds of body fat. It is not a perfect therapy, and everyone is not capable of completely transforming their lives after surgery. Our society is very understanding when orthopedic patients require a revision years after their knee or hip replacement and should be equally understanding of those patients who suffer weight regain after Bariatric Surgery and need a revision procedure down the road.

CHAPTER TEN
PREPARING FOR SURGERY

Preparing for weight loss surgery requires work on many fronts. The emotional, nutritional, medical and financial demands of weight loss surgery require preparation and forethought. The biggest "red flag" in my practice is when a new patient considering surgery informs me that he has been thinking about the surgery for a few weeks now and wants to know how soon he can get an operative date. Successful preparation for surgery requires months and often years of careful consideration and planning in order to take every step possible to ensure success. Many patients rely on the experience and advice of friends to guide them through the process, but this is often not enough to ensure success and frequently leads to conflicting advice. Good preparation requires honest conversations with your primary care physician and surgeon, research using quality resources and a healthy dose of soul searching.

Finding a Bariatric Surgeon

Most prospective weight loss surgery patients think that the most important criteria in choosing a Weight Loss Surgeon is surgical skill and safety. Thankfully, most surgeons who perform over 100 Bariatric procedures per year have an excellent safety record. While there are always a few surgeons that have an unnecessarily high complication rate, my observation of my peers is that the overwhelming majority of high-volume Bariatric surgeons are very competent and skilled. The chance that your choice of surgeon will result in you suffering a complication that a more skilled surgeon would have avoided is less than 2%-3%.

If finding the surgeon in your town with the absolute lowest complication rate is your top priority, you may struggle to find reliable data you can use to make your decision. Postoperative complication rates are poorly tracked and rarely made public. However, one interesting observation is that surgeons who are more humble often have lower complication rates[218].

Surgeons have a reputation for being arrogant and uncaring. I've certainly met a few who fit this description. But, the most skilled surgeons that I've known are also the most down to earth and humble. Surgery requires technical skill, but even more importantly, good judgment and a realistic assessment of what can and can't be accomplished in the operating room. Even the most skilled surgeons have complications. After 14 years of practice, I've had a few patients who have had a long and rocky course after their weight loss surgery. Complications are very difficult for most surgeons to deal with emotionally, and when they do occur, there are two ways to approach them. The best and most humble surgeons that I've met will review every detail of the surgery, talk to their colleagues about how they could have handled it differently, review the scientific literature for new techniques to avoid this problem going forward and come up with a plan to ensure that it doesn't happen again. Arrogant surgeons will often blame the complication on some external, uncontrollable force and learn nothing. Arrogant surgeons continue to make the same mistakes over and over again. If you want to find a skilled surgeon, look for someone who is experienced and well recommended, but also humble, down to earth and willing to listen to your story.

If you are undergoing a revision surgery or are particularly high risk due to your weight or medical history, surgical skill definitely matters by more than just a few percentage points. Finding the most skilled surgeon is often not straight forward since complication rates are typically not made public and the few registries that exist are difficult if not impossible to interpret accurately. Often the busiest or most popular surgeon in town is not the most skilled.

In my experience, there are two different types of Bariatric Surgeons: 1) surgeons who perform lots of different surgeries, including Bariatric procedures and 2) obesity specialists who perform lots of Bariatric surgeries. Determining the difference is usually not difficult. If your surgeon spends little time talking about nutrition and exercise and is quick to pass that responsibility off to the nutritionist or exercise specialist, you're speaking to a surgeon who knows how to do Bariatric operations. If your surgeon takes a detailed weight and dietary history, asks about your expectations after surgery and spends a good deal of time discussing the importance of good nutrition and exercise, then you've found an obesity specialist. While many programs have nutritionists and exercise specialists who are excellent at what they do, I believe that a Bariatric Surgeon should know as much about these topics and be as equally invested in your lifestyle changes as he or she is in the surgery.

Most importantly, you should feel that you can trust your surgeon to help you make the best decision about your body. You should feel confident that your surgeon will be there for you after surgery and not just pass you off to the nutritionist if you're not meeting your weight loss goals. When you come in for your appointment, ask others who are waiting if they are seeing the same surgeon and what their experience has been.

There is also a significant group of Bariatric Surgeons who only perform Sleeve Gastrectomy. Performing a Sleeve Gastrectomy is relatively straightforward and does not require the surgical skill that performing a Gastric Bypass safely does. If you go to see a surgeon who only performs Sleeve Gastrectomy procedures, then you may not get the most unbiased and balanced evaluation. Even if you are certain that you only want a Sleeve Gastrectomy, you should still see a surgeon who is able to perform both procedures to confirm that you are not ignoring important factors like significant heartburn or a large hiatal hernia that could result in long term complications.

Ideally, you should find a surgeon within a relatively short drive. Remember, you will likely have 10-12 appointments with your surgeon over your lifetime, so a two hour drive each way could become problematic. With the advent of telemedicine, this may become less important since most of these appointments with your surgeon and his or her team lend themselves to telemedicine. I would caution you against selecting a surgeon simply because they work in a hospital system that you're familiar with. The transfer of records between physician offices is typically a simple matter so your surgeon should have little problem obtaining all of the necessary medical records. Also, your time in the hospital will likely be only a day or two. It is very unlikely that you'll need your cardiologist, pulmonologist or internist on standby after surgery - significant heart or lung problems are very uncommon after weight loss surgery.

Insurance Coverage

Obtaining insurance coverage for Bariatric surgery is often the most difficult and frustrating part of the entire process[219]. Some insurance companies make it very easy for their enrollees to undergo Bariatric Surgery, others make it nearly impossible. Talk to the surgeon's team and ask if they frequently have trouble getting authorization from your insurance company.

Most insurance companies require a period of pre-operative, physician supervised weight loss[220]. Often, patients are referred to their primary care doctor for these visits, however some programs, like mine, will offer the counselling through their practice. Some patients look at the physician supervised weight loss period as nothing more than a box that must be checked in order to satisfy the insurance company's requirements. However, these months preceding the surgery can be an excellent opportunity to prepare for life after surgery. I work with my patients to make one, meaningful change to their diet each month. After a few months, patients have increased their vegetable intake, decreased their sugar intake, eliminated all sugar sweetened beverages, limited artificial sweeteners and made many of the changes that are required for success after surgery.

Most insurance companies also require a psychological evaluation prior to surgery. This requirement is not grounded in solid scientific evidence, but it remains a staple of the preoperative requirements for nearly every insurance plan in the United States[221]. The psychological evaluation typically consists of answering hundreds of bubble sheeted questions designed to determine if you exhibit impulsive or compulsive behaviors, suffer from eating disorders, are suicidal, have a substance abuse disorder or exhibit any other tendencies believed to pose a risk to your postoperative success. Usually, the evaluation can be accomplished in an afternoon, however, many psychologists will require several follow up visits.

I've noticed tremendous variation in the quality of pre-operative psychological evaluations. Many patients report the experience as very helpful and use it to establish a relationship with a therapist that they can lean on after surgery to help deal with postoperative emotions. However, a number of patients often report that the evaluation was tedious, unnecessarily long and expensive. Again, the staff at your Bariatric Surgeon's office can be very useful in helping you determine which psychologist you should see. There are also several online services that will complete an evaluation over the phone. While I question the value of what often amounts to a short phone call, I also recognize that not all prospective patients have a clinical need for the psychological evaluation that their insurance company requires. For those patients without clinically significant depression, a history of a substance abuse disorder or suicide attempts who are generally doing just fine in the rest of their life, but just need help losing weight, an online service may be your most convenient option.

If you are denied insurance approval for your Bariatric procedure, don't panic, you still have several options available to you. The first step is to determine why you were denied coverage - the insurance company must provide a reason. Often, there is a clear request for additional evaluation or documentation and the denial will be overturned after this information is submitted. Occasionally, the reasons are more difficult to remedy and a peer to peer evaluation is required in which your surgeon speaks to a physician who works for the insurance company. In my experience, peer to peer evaluations are less likely to be successful than simple requests for additional documentation.

There are several insurance companies that set requirements that are nearly impossible for most patients to satisfy. Many patients respond to denials from these insurance companies with appeals that Bariatric Surgery will improve their health and prevent or treat heart disease or diabetes. While this is certainly true, when appealing to insurance companies for coverage, this fact is, unfortunately, completely ignored.

Health insurance is a legal contract between the insurance company and you, the beneficiary. This legal contract explicitly states which services are covered, and which services are excluded. For those covered services, the contract states what steps must be fulfilled before the insurance company will agree to pay for the health care services. This is a legal contract, so moral or medical appeals will be ignored. The hard truth about health insurance is that appeals for coverage based on your health are considered with as much importance as a plea to your mortgage lender that you can't make your payment this month because you're short on cash.

Because this is a legal contract, not a moral obligation, your appeal must be based on satisfying the requirements stated in the contract, not on the ways the surgery will benefit you. There is a very helpful and fair company that can assist you in your appeal that is run by a passionate Bariatric Surgery patient, Walter Lindstrom. Walter's company can be found online at www.wlsappeals.com and has extensive experience successfully battling insurance companies for weight loss surgery coverage approvals. The website also offers a wealth of information about insurance coverage for Bariatric Surgery.

While most insurance policies cover Bariatric Surgery, there are many people whose policy specifically excludes coverage. This unfortunate group still has options, but it can get expensive. As of 2019, there are policies on healthcare.gov that cover Bariatric Surgery, however this will vary from state to state. Often there is a high co-pay with these policies and a waiting period, but it is usually a little less expensive than paying for the entire procedure out of pocket.

For those who elect to pay for their procedure out of pocket, there are several companies who offer financing. Most commonly, people use Care Credit (carecredit.com) and Prosper Healthcare (prosperhealthcare.com) to finance their procedure over 3-5 years. A Sleeve Gastrectomy typically costs between $12,000 to $16,000 and a Gastric Bypass procedure is usually $3,000 to $4,000 more. Choosing to self-pay for your surgery also limits the number of surgeons that you can choose from since many hospitals do not have affordable programs set up.

Many patients look to medical tourism options when exploring self-pay surgery since other countries, most commonly Mexico, offer procedures for less than half the cost offered in the United States. For some patients, this is a reasonable decision. If you are relatively healthy, have not had extensive abdominal surgery in the past and are considering a Sleeve Gastrectomy, it is likely that you'll have a good outcome if you are able to find a quality center outside the country. If you have multiple medical problems, have had previous abdominal surgery or are pursuing a Gastric Bypass, you should not pursue medical tourism.

The decision to leave the country for your procedure should not be made lightly. In the United States, you are guaranteed a minimum standard of quality in every hospital because of the regulation of healthcare facilities. Mexico does not provide this same degree of regulation and basic principles like proper sterile technique or appropriate training of all health care providers is not guaranteed. Despite this, there are centers in Mexico that do provide quality care and are reasonable options for those who can't obtain insurance coverage and can't afford US prices. Differentiating quality centers from facilities that don't meet the most basic standards can be difficult. If you are considering this option, do your research first and don't hesitate to back out at the last minute if it does not feel safe, even if it means that you will lose money.

If you have complications after a self-pay operation, this can be financially devastating. For those patients who have health insurance, but do not have Bariatric Surgery coverage, your health insurance plan may pay for coverage of complications, even if they don't cover the surgery. For those that don't have insurance coverage, if you are unfortunate to suffer a significant complication, you can find yourself severely in debt and your only recourse may be to declare bankruptcy. Leavitt Risk Partners (www.leavittriskpartners.com) offers insurance for complications after self-pay surgery. While they provide an important service, the amount of coverage is limited and will not be enough to pay for a catastrophic complication.

Just as obesity is a chronic disease that develops over decades, the road to weight loss surgery can take several years. If you are faced with insurance obstacles that seem insurmountable, or the self-pay option is completely unaffordable, you may have to put aside your plan for surgery for now. Insurance plans are constantly changing, and a market is developing for lower cost self-pay procedures. Don't despair if you are unable to proceed with surgery. Perhaps this setback is providing you an opportunity to focus more on your lifestyle habits, making you a better prepared patient for next year when your insurance coverage changes.

CHAPTER ELEVEN
EATING BEFORE SURGERY

Insurance companies require most patients to participate in a three- or six-month period of monthly visits with a physician to document that their weight loss is not amenable to dieting and exercise alone[220]. In my practice, I work with patients to slowly implement my Pound of Cure[222] program over these months, rather than impose a radical, often difficult to follow change immediately. Each month, I provide one simple rule that the patient will follow in order to slowly improve his or her diet. After five months, the resulting diet resembles an ideal post-operative diet.

Most people devote their energy toward resisting the tempting, set point raising foods that cause weight gain. My approach to nutrition is focused on eating more of the foods that drive weight loss, rather than resisting processed foods. Many practices push low calorie prepared meals, protein shakes and bars and emphasize a "protein first" lifelong approach to nutrition. Instead, I encourage my patients to focus more on unprocessed, whole foods. I believe that patients should focus on a lifelong "produce first" approach, rather than consuming large amounts of processed protein drinks and bars.

Each month, I encourage patients to learn how to make one or two simple, easy to prepare meals that represent the change we're trying to make that month. By the end of the six-month process, they will know how to make nearly a dozen new meals that can replace the standard, processed food that most of us prepare for ourselves. Many patients think that they can wait until after the surgery to start making these changes. This is not a good strategy. After surgery, you should be able to focus on your recovery and adjusting to the slower pace of eating and smaller portion sizes. Trying to learn new recipes and recover from surgery at the same time can be overwhelming and cause unnecessary stress.

Month 1: One Pound of Vegetables (or more)

Without question, the healthiest foods on the planet are vegetables[223]. The healthiest of all are green leafy vegetables like spinach and kale, followed closely by green, solid vegetables like broccoli, asparagus, celery and cucumbers. Solid, non-green vegetables like carrots and cauliflower are still excellent sources of nutrition and should be eaten liberally but, on average, have less nutrition than green vegetables[224]. While beans and colorful, starchy vegetables like squash, sweet potatoes and beets are excellent, I typically exclude them from being counted toward your daily tally. To be counted as part of your pound for the day, vegetables cannot be eaten with any creamy or oily dressings or dips.

I start with vegetables since they represent the backbone of a healthy diet. As you start to incorporate more vegetables into your diet, you will find yourself naturally making better food choices throughout the day[225]. Many patients start eating their pound of vegetables by focusing on raw carrots, celery and broccoli. While this is a good starting point, truly incorporating vegetables into your diet means making them a part of every meal, rather than eating them only as a snack. I encourage patients to get creative with their vegetable dishes and to search out new recipes that use vegetables in interesting and often delicious ways. Long term lifestyle change does not mean giving up your enjoyment of food, it means finding different types of food to enjoy.

Vegetables – A thorough but not complete list

artichokes	cucumber	peppers, red
arugula	daikon	peppers, yellow
asparagus	eggplant	radicchio
bamboo shoot	endive	radishes
beans, green	fennel	red leaf lettuce
beans, yellow	kale	romaine lettuce
bok-choy	kohlrabi	scallions
Boston lettuce	mushrooms	shallots
broccoli	okra	soybeans
broccoflower	onion	spinach
Brussels sprouts	parsley	squash
cabbage	peas, black eyed	Swiss chard
carrots	peas, green	tomato
cauliflower	peas, snap	turnips
celery	peas, snow	water chestnuts
chickpeas	peas, split	zucchini
collard greens	peppers, green	

Month 2: Say goodbye to Sugar and Artificial Sweeteners. Instead, eat lots of fruit.

Human beings are hardwired to like sweet foods. This is not an unfortunate side effect; a preference for sweet foods offers a distinct evolutionary advantage. Our caveman ancestors obtained a significant portion of their calories by foraging for foods - the bounty of meat from a successful hunt was more likely an occasional treat, rather than a daily staple[226]. Foraging carries a risk of mistaking a poisonous plant for its edible twin. Cavemen dedicated a significant amount of energy toward learning which foods could be safely eaten and which should be avoided. In nature, there are no foods that contain fructose that are poisonous. Fructose's sweet taste is a simple and reliable method to identify a food that is safe to eat. Children carried the highest risk of accidental poisoning due to their small size and lack of experience with foraging, explaining why children are particularly interested in sweets over all other foods[227].

Thankfully, accidental poisoning is a rare event in our modern world, however, our inborn preference and drive toward sweet foods persist. Many diet plans unfairly vilify fruit due to its sugar content and restrict or limit it. Many patients are surprised when I encourage them to eat as much fruit as they possibly can both before and after surgery, even higher sugar varieties like bananas, grapes, mangoes and cherries.

First, there are no studies that I am aware of that demonstrate that increased fruit intake causes weight gain. However, there are many studies that demonstrate the opposite[228,229,230]. Second, when we look at life after surgery, it's important that we draw our battle lines appropriately. Success after surgery is not dependant on reducing sugar intake, it's dependent on reducing **refined** sugar intake. This is a battle against cherry pie, not cherries and banana splits, not bananas. Making your postoperative diet too restrictive is a recipe for failure. It's important to set yourself up for success by satisfying your prehistoric drive for sweets with fruit to ensure that you don't give in to temptation and eat foods that contain refined sugar.

Eliminating refined sugar from your diet seems like a daunting task at first, but after a few weeks, it becomes quite manageable. Once you are through the first week or two of your sugar detox, you will find that fruit easily satisfies your sweet cravings and you can limit your intake of refined sweets to once a week or less.

Sugar sweetened beverages, especially soda-pop, require particular attention. Our body has two separate methods for regulating hunger and thirst. Food makes us less hungry, and water makes us less thirsty, but food does not address our thirst and water does not address our appetite. There are a few exceptions to this rule. Watery food like watermelon can reduce our thirst and thick liquids like protein shakes will reduce our hunger. However, sugar containing beverages are thin liquids that address our thirst but have a very small impact on our hunger[231]. The result is that the calories in sugar sweetened beverages like soda-pop, fruit juice, sports drinks, sweetened coffee drinks, sweet tea, lemonade and fruit punch slide in under the radar of our metabolic thermostat[232]. Our metabolic thermostat works very aggressively to match our calorie expenditure to our calorie consumption but is not dialed into the calories in thin liquids. This defect is understandable since there are no thin liquids that exist naturally and contain calories.

Because calories from sugar sweetened beverages do not impact our hunger, they don't trigger the metabolic adjustments that occur when the same number of calories are consumed as food. A 12 ounce can of Pepsi contains 150 calories. If you consume one can daily and these calories aren't accounted for by your metabolic thermostat and are stored, rather than burned, these 150 calories daily can result in as much as 15 lbs of weight gain per year[ii]. When I see patients in the office who report primary weight gain (not regain) of more than 10 lbs. per year, there are only a few factors that can drive this much weight gain and sugar sweetened beverages is at the top of this list. Sugar sweetened beverages are tightly linked to weight gain, obesity and diabetes[233,234,235,236]. **Success after surgery is not possible without eliminating these drinks from your diet forever.** When I see patients who have regained a significant amount of weight after surgery, sugar sweetened beverages are a common culprit.

[ii] Assuming 3,500 kCal in one pound of body fat

Artificially sweetened beverages are not nearly as fattening as sugar containing beverages[237], however they present a much more significant threat to your long-term success than most people appreciate. Since the majority of dieting advice focuses on either calorie or carbohydrate restriction, artificial sweeteners have been given a free pass[238]. Recently, there have been many well publicized scientific studies that demonstrate that artificial sweeteners play a significant role in weight gain, despite not containing calories[239,240]. There are two mechanisms by which these substances contribute to weight gain.

The first way that artificial sweeteners cause weight gain is by hijacking your tastebuds so they are only sensitive to super sweet foods[241]. On a sweetness scale, artificial sweeteners are much sweeter than fruit. The result of consuming large amounts of artificially sweetened foods and drinks is that fruit is no longer perceived as sweet, increasing your drive for sweeter foods like those that contain refined sugar. This process is known as "taste adaptation" and explains why those who consume artificially sweetened foods and beverages also struggle to avoid foods that contain real sugar[242]. As you progress through this month of sugar detoxification, you will begin to appreciate the sweetness of fruit as your taste buds adjust to naturally sweet foods. Many patients report to me that they cannot believe how sweet the apples, peaches or cherries are this year, compared to last year. It's likely that this is not due to a good year in the orchard, but rather a new-found ability to taste and appreciate fruit after eliminating artificial sweeteners from their diet.

The second way that artificial sweeteners cause weight gain becomes clear only after we recognize that it's our metabolic thermostat that drives weight gain and loss, rather than simply excess calories. As we've discussed, our body has an extremely tight system of regulating our calorie expenditure based on our calorie consumption. When we dig into the physiology of how this happens, we find that taste plays a major role in the inner workings of our metabolic thermostat. Our sweet taste buds let our brain know that a load of sugar is coming, triggering our pancreas to release sugar metabolizing enzymes and allowing the rest of our body to feel comfortable that food is present so our metabolism can run at its full capacity. Artificial sweeteners trigger our sweet tastebuds but don't deliver the calorie load that our body is expecting. As a result, our normally tightly regulated system of matching calorie expenditure to calorie consumption begins to break down[243]. Our metabolism loses its ability to respond appropriately to other sweet foods with refined and natural sugar. The net result is a shift in your metabolic thermostat toward weight gain[244].

Stevia deserves an extra comment since it is frequently misunderstood. Because Stevia is marketed as a natural sweetener, many people think that it does not cause the same negative effects that other artificial sweeteners do. This is not true, Stevia is as dangerous as the blue, pink and yellow artificial sweeteners. While a stevia plant does represent a natural, unprocessed food, the white powder that you put in your coffee is not natural. **Artificial sweeteners that come from refining a stevia plant are no more natural of a sweetener than the table sugar that comes from refining a sugar cane plant.**

Month 3: Eliminate processed junk food and replace it with lots of nuts.

Processed, high calorie junk food is everywhere these days. Most of us think about chips, cookies and fast food when the words "junk food" are mentioned, however, there are many other foods that are equally processed and fattening. If we label all refined or processed food as "junk", we should include most granola bars, breakfast cereals, yogurts, frozen meals (even the low-calorie ones), white breads and rolls and most pastas. When we use this stricter definition of junk food, most Americans derive around 60% of their daily calories from junk food[245].

Junk foods consist primarily of processed carbohydrates that are rapidly absorbed by your intestine shortly after you eat them. The carbohydrates that exist in beans, vegetables, fruit, whole grains and nuts are more slowly absorbed. The rate at which carbohydrates are absorbed determines how likely they are to be converted to fat and stored. You may have heard the term "glycemic index" used as an explanation of whether a food is fattening. The glycemic index is measured by checking people's blood sugars after eating certain foods. Those foods with a low glycemic index result in a modest increase in your blood sugar, while high glycemic index foods cause a rapid increase[246].

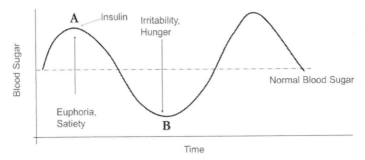

Figure 18 - Your blood sugar after eating high glycemic index foods

The graphic above shows the cyclic changes in blood sugar that occur after eating high glycemic index junk food. Shortly after eating the junk, your blood sugar goes up rapidly until you reach point A. When your blood sugar is a little high, you typically feel full and satisfied. However, your metabolism responds to a high blood sugar by releasing Insulin, a hormone that works to bring your blood sugar back to a normal level. Insulin doesn't just magically reduce your blood sugar levels – it lowers the amount of sugar in your blood by driving the sugar out of your blood and into your liver and fat cells where it will be eventually converted to body fat.

Rapid rises in blood sugar result in the release of lots of insulin. A rapid release of Insulin often overshoots its target resulting in a low blood sugar level an hour or so after eating (point B). Low blood sugar causes hunger and irritability triggering you to, of course, eat more junk food. This cycle often occurs many times each day and leaves the patient wondering why they struggle with difficult to control food cravings[247].

The solution to managing this roller coaster ride is not willpower, it's to not get on the ride in the first place[248]. During month 3, I challenge my patients to eliminate all junk food. Giving up these foods is usually not difficult for most of my patients, until they find themselves short of time and hungry. Junk food is not particularly good tasting, it's just extremely convenient. Grab a buck, walk down the hall to the vending machine and, a granola bar is delivered. You go back to your busy life, and without a conscious thought, you devour the granola bar. Often, the only thing that reminds you that you just ate it is the empty wrapper in the garbage can.

Thankfully, there is a food that is widely available (even in most vending machines) that is completely healthy, delicious, affordable and will not cause weight gain. While nuts and seeds are often vilified as being high in fat and calories, there is an abundance of literature that demonstrates that increasing your daily consumption of nuts often leads to weight loss, not weight gain as most would think[249,250,251].

There is lots of discussion about which type of nut or seed is the healthiest, however, the actual differences are negligible. Even peanuts, which are technically legumes, not nuts, make an excellent snack. The important factor in the healthfulness of nuts and seeds is the preparation. Nut and seed preparations can be categorized into four different groups.

Raw (also known as natural) - This is the healthiest preparation; however, the nuts and seeds lack the crunch that is often necessary to replace junk food. They are not baked, and nothing is added to them. They are harvested, shelled and then sold. Raw nuts and seeds rarely come salted, however, if you like, feel free to add a little salt and toast them.

Dry Roasted - These are nuts or seeds that are essentially toasted, but do not have anything added to them during the cooking process. They come in salted & unsalted varieties. Again, feel free to select the salted versions without guilt. Eliminating junk food will result in such a significant decrease in your daily sodium intake, a little salted, dry roasted nuts or seeds will still ensure that you are consuming much less sodium than before.

Roasted - Roasted nuts are coated in oil and then heated. Roasted nuts can easily be differentiated from dry roasted preparations by looking at the list of ingredients. Dry Roasted nuts will list only nuts and salt in the ingredient list, while roasted nuts or seeds will also list oil. Often the oil comes from the same nut or seed. For instance, peanuts are often roasted in peanut oil and sunflower seeds are roasted in sunflower oil. Nut oils are very heat sensitive. When nut oils are heated, they can transform into trans-fats. Trans-fats cause heart disease and weight gain and there is even legislation that prevents them from being used in foods. However, this legislation only factors in the original ingredients, not the by-products of the cooking process. Because of the added oil and potential for exposure to trans-fats, *roasted nuts should be avoided if possible[252].*

Roasted and sweetened – These are roasted nuts or seeds with a flavoring that contains sugar or other sweeteners. Honey, Barbecue and Spicy preparations often have sugar added, making these oiled and sweetened nuts or seeds as dangerous as the junk food you are trying to replace.

Month 3 marks another big step in cleaning up your diet. By the end of the third month, you will be eating a pound or more of vegetables, minimal refined sugar or artificial sweeteners, lots of fruit, nuts and seeds and very little junk food. You will be well on the road to the healthy diet that will ensure that your weight loss surgery results in a life free of obesity.

Month 4 - Eat lots of colorful starchy vegetables and cut down on grains and low nutrient, colorless vegetables like corn and potatoes

America's obsession with low-carbohydrate diets has unfairly denigrated many wonderful foods that are critical to your long-term success. While processed carbohydrates must be avoided, carbs that come from colorful, starchy vegetables make excellent choices. Sweet potatoes, beets and squash are excellent foods that can be consumed comfortably within a few weeks of surgery[253]. Eating large amounts of colorful, starchy vegetables will also decrease your desire for grains, potatoes and corn that will compromise your long-term success.

Whole grains have received lots of positive press, but those who encourage the consumption of large amounts of unprocessed grains are often doing so as part of a business plan, rather than because of good science. The Oldways Whole Grains Council appears to be a non-profit consumer watchdog group put in place to help people choose healthy foods that are made from unprocessed grains. Their stamp of approval has been placed on over 10,000 different food products and adorns many cereal boxes that are loaded with sugar and artificial flavors. It should come as no surprise to learn that this "consumer watchdog group" is heavily funded by the food industry[254].

While whole grain foods contain lots of fiber, their health benefits can only be demonstrated when they are compared to processed grains like white bread and pasta[255,256]. There is very little scientific evidence that demonstrates that adding whole grain foods to your diet improves your health. I think the switch from processed grains like white bread and pasta to whole grain alternatives is like changing from full tar cigarettes to low tar cigarettes. While the low tar versions may be slightly less toxic, they do not present a suitable alternative to quitting smoking altogether.

Many postoperative patients are able to incorporate colorful starchy vegetables into their diet within a week or two of surgery. Well-cooked sweet potatoes and squash go down very easily and provide calories and vitamins that help to ease your recovery. I recommend eating these foods frequently throughout the day starting in the second week after surgery.

Good Colorful, Starchy Vegetables	*Bad* Grains and grain-like vegetables	*Ugly* Processed Grains
Beets	*Buckwheat*	*White Bread*
Squash	*Brown Rice*	*White Rice*
Sweet Potatoes	*Corn*	*White Pasta*
Turnips	*Millet*	*Instant Oatmeal*
Yams	*Oats*	
	Popcorn	
	Quinoa	
	White Potatoes	
	Whole grain breads	

To simplify my patients' understanding of carbohydrates, I break them down into "the good," "the bad," and "the ugly." Foods that are in the good category can be eaten liberally, even in large portions without concern for weight regain after surgery. Those in the "bad" category have more potential to cause weight regain and have to be consumed with care[257]. I've found that patients who have had a particularly strong response to surgery or are exercising regularly can incorporate foods in the "bad" category into their diet without concern for weight regain. Those patients who have struggled with their postoperative weight loss or are sedentary after surgery should be very careful with these foods since even small amounts can cause weight regain.

Foods in the "ugly" category must be avoided completely by all postoperative patients. These "white" foods will threaten even the most successful postoperative patient's weight loss[258]. Thankfully, there are many delicious substitutes for pasta, bread and white rice that make avoiding these foods possible. There are several brands of pasta made entirely from beans, or a flour made from beans (usually chickpeas). These are often found in the gluten free aisle but differ from the other gluten free products since they are made from beans, rather than other gluten free grains like rice. Off all the bread substitutes, I think that the sprouted grain breads like Ezekiel make the best choice. However, they still contain wheat and may contribute to weight gain in some. An even better alternative is to convert your sandwich into a salad by replacing the bread with a green leafy vegetable. This works well for most sandwiches (turkey, ham, chicken and hamburgers), but not for all. I'm not sure that a peanut butter and jelly salad would be appealing. Finally, white rice can be replaced with "riced" cauliflower that is similar in taste and texture.

Month 5 - Eat less meat and more beans

I try to never use the "V" word in my practice because I find that the idea of vegetarianism is unacceptable to most people. I am not a practicing vegetarian and have no plans to become one and I fully understand people's reluctance to not commit to a meat-free lifestyle.

However, you do not have to avoid meat altogether in order to gain most of the health benefits that vegetarianism offers. Vegetarianism is usually thought of as a social movement to draw attention toward animal rights and the cruelty of raising animals just for food. However, in recent years, vegetarianism as a health movement has gained traction after several important studies showed significantly lower rates of heart disease and cancer in vegetarians[259,260].

If we look at the consumption of meat as a health decision, rather than a moral one, vegetarianism becomes a spectrum, rather than an absolute decision. If the decision not to eat meat is made for social reasons, one single bite of meat is murder and cannot be tolerated. However, if this decision is made for health reasons, then one single bite is insignificant. It is the daily consumption of large amounts of meat that must be avoided and any decision to eat less meat is a step in the right direction. Meat has been tightly linked to diabetes[261], heart disease[262] and, contrary to what the Ketogenic or Paleo diet supporters will tell you, eating large amounts of meat will lead to weight gain[263,264].

I encourage my patients to limit their intake of animal protein to two 3-4 ounce servings per day. 3-4 ounces of meat is approximately the size of a deck of cards, so, for most, this change will represent a reduction in the amount of animal protein that they consume. Those who want to reduce their consumption further are encouraged to do so.

All food that comes from animals is considered "meat." Fish, chicken, eggs and dairy products all exhibit a similar nutritional effect to beef and pork[265]. Many people believe that the type of meat that you consume is the most important measure of its health effects. For instance, most people believe that eating beef is much less healthy than eating chicken. In truth, exactly the opposite may be true. The way an animal is raised will greatly impact the health impact of the meat. For instance, beef that comes from a cow that was raised organically, without hormones or antibiotics and allowed to roam free and eat grass has less of a negative impact on your health when compared to chicken that was genetically engineered to grow quickly, given large amounts of antibiotics and fed a highly processed diet[266].

When it comes to animal protein, purchasing small amounts of a higher quality, organically raised meat is an excellent strategy. The price is often twice that of conventional animal products, but you will be eating far less, neutralizing the cost difference.

There are several good techniques out there that help you reduce your meat consumption significantly without feeling overly restricted. The VB6 movement encourages people to avoid eating any animal products before 6pm and is a simple way to limit your daily meat consumption significantly[267]. "Weekday veganism" takes a similar approach and encourages people to avoid meat from Monday through Friday, but on the weekends when many people have gatherings that are centered around food and eating, you can feel free to indulge[268]. Adopting either one of these strategies to prevent weight regain after surgery is strongly encouraged.

After Bariatric Surgery, many patients lose their taste for meat and are not able to consume it comfortably for up to a year. This puts patients in a difficult position as they try to increase their protein intake. Even those patients who are able to keep animal protein down comfortably within a few weeks of surgery are often only able to eat a few bites which contributes little to their total protein intake.

Instead, I encourage patients to eat lots of vegetable protein after surgery, specifically, beans and nuts. These foods are much more comfortable to eat than animal sources of protein, so postoperative patients may actually be able to consume more protein through beans and nuts since they can eat much more of them.

Beans contain a substantial amount of protein as well as loads of dietary fiber. Even more importantly, regular consumption of beans is associated with lower blood pressure, lower body weight, smaller waist circumference and a lower incidence of diabetes[269]. Despite their high carbohydrate intake, beans may be one of the best foods for diabetics to eat[270].

Protein from yogurt lies somewhere in between animal and vegetable protein in terms of its health effects. Yogurt contains a favorable mix of bacteria that has been linked to weight loss (especially if you also eat lots of fruit)[271]. Other dairy products like cheese or milk do not demonstrate the same weight loss benefits[272]. Yogurt can be easily consumed within a few days of surgery and contains reasonable amounts of protein, especially Greek yogurt. I strongly encourage patients to purchase plain yogurt and mix it with fruit in a blender, rather than purchasing pre-packaged flavored yogurts since they almost always contain added sugar or artificial sweeteners.

Most practices encourage the prolonged use of protein shakes after surgery, while I do not. I find that many patients cannot tolerate the artificially sweetened and flavored protein shakes after surgery. When patients complain that they can't tolerate their postoperative shakes, I quickly move them onto yogurt smoothies which contain almost equivalent amounts of protein without the artificial additives. Often, these smoothies are well tolerated, while the shakes cause nausea.

Many patients find the changes in Month 5 are not nearly as difficult as they initially thought they would be. Moving to smaller amounts of higher quality animal protein and increasing your consumption of beans and yogurt is an important step toward success after surgery.

Month 6: Your preoperative diet

In the final month, I prepare the patient for his or her preoperative, fasting diet. The preoperative diet differs significantly from the Pound of Cure style of eating that we've been working on. The Pound of Cure eating style is designed as a way of eating that can be maintained life long and prevents weight regain after surgery. The preoperative diet is designed to induce rapid, short term weight loss. This weight loss can't be maintained over the long run[273], but this is irrelevant as you approach surgery.

The goal of the preoperative diet is to trigger rapid weight loss over a short period of time. When you lose weight quickly, it depletes the liver of fat which makes the surgery easier and safer to perform[274]. The most effective way to lose weight quickly is by severely restricting your calorie intake. The pre-operative diet limits your calorie intake to around 800 calories per day with very little carbohydrate intake. The easiest way to do this is through the use of meal replacement protein shakes.

There are hundreds of brands of protein shakes available, however, despite the marketing claims, they are incredibly similar to each other. The most common source of protein in these shakes comes from whey which is derived from milk. Despite this, those patients with lactose intolerance are usually able to tolerate whey protein well since the lactose is removed during the processing. Some of the less expensive or "vegan" shakes use soy protein. Soy can stimulate estrogen receptors[275] (which are present in both men and women) and large doses can create hormonal irregularities that are undesirable in the days leading up to surgery. Recently, shakes with pea or peanut protein have become popular but probably do not convey a significant advantage over whey protein shakes. These "vegan" shakes are typically two to three times as expensive as those that use whey protein. Whatever protein shake you choose should contain 15-20 grams of protein, less than 3 grams of sugar and contain less than 200 calories each.

I also allow unlimited calorie free drinks (anything less than 10 calories per serving) on the pre-operative diet which goes directly against my teaching of the dangers of artificial sweeteners. The preoperative diet is difficult to follow and is only a short-term program. I've found that eliminating sugar free drinks makes this diet exceptionally difficult to follow and decreases compliance. Again, the goal of the preoperative diet is to lose weight quickly over a short period of time in preparation for surgery.

Finally, I allow unlimited green vegetables (except avocadoes) on the preoperative diet. You can use unlimited seasonings and spices, but no butter or oil. As we've discussed, vegetables facilitate weight loss and may help your body from entering starvation mode during the severe calorie restriction imposed by the diet.

For some patients, tight compliance with the preoperative diet is critical to their safety. For other patients, it is much less important. A very small percentage of patients have severe fatty liver disease that interferes with the safety of the operation. Men, high BMI patients, diabetics and those whose weight is concentrated in their belly, rather than their buttocks and thighs are more difficult to operate on. A preoperative diet, often for two weeks or more is critical to safe surgery[276]. For those patients who don't fall into the higher risk group, I limit the preoperative diet to a less restrictive program, often for only one week. In the lower risk patients, I also allow them to follow the Pound of Cure "Metabolic Reset Diet" described in detail in my first book.

I've listed the instructions I provide for my patients but ask that you defer to your surgeon if he or she uses a different pre-operative diet.

All Men (regardless of BMI) and Women with a BMI >50

- Four Protein Shakes every day (not to exceed 100 grams of protein daily)
- Every morning 1 sugar free fiber drink (Metamucil or similar) if necessary to maintain normal bowel habits
- Take a Multivitamin daily (Bariatric vitamins are acceptable)
- Unlimited Calorie Free Liquids

- Unlimited green vegetables (except avocadoes)
- Start 2 weeks prior to your surgical date (or longer if instructed)

All Women with a BMI <50

- Two Protein Shakes every day (one for breakfast, one for lunch)
- A healthy, low carbohydrate dinner (<400 calories)
- Every morning 1 sugar free fiber drink (Metamucil or similar) if necessary to maintain normal bowel habits
- Take a Multivitamin daily (Bariatric vitamins are acceptable)
- Unlimited Calorie Free Liquids
- Unlimited green vegetables (except avocadoes)
- Start 1 week prior to your surgical date
- It is acceptable to follow the Metabolic Reset Diet instead

CHAPTER TWELVE
EMOTIONAL PREPARATION

There is no "one size fits all" advice for emotionally preparing for weight loss surgery. For some, weight loss surgery marks an important emotional milestone in their life, while others are much less emotionally invested. However, everyone who chooses to have weight loss surgery has some expectations about how this surgery will impact their life.

People's motivations for choosing weight loss surgery vary tremendously and any emotional planning must take the underlying factors that are driving your decision into account. I've listed some of the most common reasons that people choose weight loss surgery below with some advice if these words strike an emotional chord.

"I'm sick of being judged because I'm overweight"

Many people decide to have weight loss surgery simply because they just don't want to spend the rest of their life overweight. Society judges those who suffer weight problems harshly and there is ample evidence that people with obesity are less successful at work, have lower self-esteem and are judged harshly by their peers and even their doctors[277]. Weight loss surgery offers an opportunity to be judged more fairly by others.

For those of you who elect surgery to remedy this discrimination, it is important to fully consider all the factors that could be causing "discrimination." My experience is that surgery does little to change your professional or close personal relationships. Those who are struggling at work may be quick to blame their lack of promotion on their boss's discrimination against them because of their weight, but it's more likely it's their job performance that's holding them back. Bad marriages often become worse after one partner undergoes weight loss surgery, while good marriages become stronger.

Friends who also struggle with their weight are often threatened when those close to them undergo weight loss surgery. Often those who suffer from obesity use close friends or family who are heavier to rationalize their own weight problems. Without you knowing it, these people in your life may use you as a standard for their own weight, telling themselves that it's not a concerning problem since they're less overweight than you. When you undergo surgery and lose weight quickly, they may no longer be able to explain away their weight problems and be forced to make some difficult assessments of their own body.

What often does change for the better after surgery is your relationship with strangers and casual acquaintances. Many people tell me they notice that others are much friendlier after surgery and, at times, postoperative patients begin to receive attention from the opposite sex. Often, this is a welcome change, but it can be uncomfortable for others.

Personal and professional relationships are complex and are just as likely to end up in worse shape after one side undergoes weight loss surgery. Those patients who look to surgery to help improve their relationships with others rarely recognize this goal. Instead, what improves much more frequently is your relationship with yourself.

"I want to have more self-esteem"

It is easy to quantify the health benefits of weight loss surgery, while the emotional gains are much harder to measure, but no less important. Patients frequently report greater confidence and happiness after surgery[278]. However, these effects vary tremendously from person to person and are hard to predict.

The difference between a desire to no longer be judged unfairly by society, and a desire for greater self-esteem is subtle, but very important. **The motivation for this surgery should come from a desire to improve yourself, not to improve how others view you**. The only thing that we can control is how we view ourselves- we cannot force others to think of us in a certain way. If you want to be a better husband or wife by being able to participate in activities that your spouse enjoys, you are likely to be very happy with your postoperative results. If you want to develop more self-confidence so you can finally end your unhealthy marriage, surgery will likely give you the boost you need to finally make this difficult decision. However, if you think weight loss surgery will make your spouse love you or respect you more, you are very likely to be let down.

These surgeries can result in a dramatic increase in your self-confidence and will likely change the way you view the world. Often this leads to a better, happier life, but other times, it reveals issues that you've used your weight as an excuse for. While most programs require an evaluation by a psychologist prior to surgery, a single evaluation is often inadequate to identify future emotional pitfalls. In my practice, I look at the initial psychological evaluation as an introduction to a trusted therapist who understands what post-weight loss surgery patients go through. While the initial evaluation is helpful, more importantly, it sets the stage for a future relationship if patients are struggling postoperatively. For those patients who already have a relationship with a psychologist, it is imperative that you discuss your motivation for surgery with your therapist and analyze your reasons for your decision.

"I'm sick of feeling sick"

If you struggle with basic daily activities like climbing steps, walking for more than a few minutes or getting on the ground to play with your children or grandchildren, you are not alone. Nearly all of my pre-operative patients report these limitations in their ability to be an active participant in their life. The good news is that weight loss surgery will dramatically improve your ability to walk, exercise, eat well, climb steps and play with your children or grandchildren[279].

Also, for those of you who know your local pharmacist by name and take many different pills or injections every day, weight loss surgery will change everything for you. Most patients are able to stop their insulin after surgery[280]. Often, postoperative patients are able to cut the number of pills that they take daily to a fraction of what they were taking preoperatively[281]. On more than one occasion, I've seen a post-surgical patient pare the number of pills they take daily from over 20 to only a daily vitamin. These changes are remarkable and add many years to your life, and, as importantly, result in a much more enjoyable life. Many of the things that you couldn't do before surgery because of your health, like travel, walking distances, swimming, living independently and spending time outdoors become possible again after surgery.

As a physician, participating in these health transformations is intensely rewarding. Every day, I am able to help patients accomplish things that I was taught in medical school were impossible. Twenty years ago, I was taught that diseases like diabetes, high blood pressure, sleep apnea, acid reflux and heart disease could only be managed with medications, but never cured. Today, I am able to prove this teaching wrong several times a week.

"I don't want to die early"

Many patients make the decision to undergo weight loss surgery out of a fear that their obesity will shorten their life. While obesity can certainly shorten your life, this isn't true for everyone who is overweight[282]. Often, I'll meet with a perfectly healthy woman in her 40's who is 100 lbs. overweight with no family history of diabetes or heart disease and no medical problems other than occasionally sore joints. Although this woman is overweight, it is very unlikely that obesity will shorten her life. Alternatively, a man in his 40's who is only 50 pounds overweight yet suffers from diabetes, high blood pressure, high cholesterol and has already had one heart attack is at great risk for a shortened life due to his obesity. Body weight or BMI as an independent measure of your risk of an early death is not a perfect determinant. For some, weight loss surgery offers a significant opportunity to add years to your life, while for others, the health benefits are minimal. For those who already suffer from obesity related medical conditions like heart disease, diabetes, high blood pressure and high cholesterol, weight loss surgery significantly reduces your risk of early death, while those who are overweight without health conditions already have a very small risk of early death that will not be significantly affected by a decision to undergo weight loss surgery[283].

Often, I find that patients will use their fear of an early death as their explanation to others for their reasoning behind their decision, while, in reality, their decisions are much more emotional and personal. This is a perfectly reasonable strategy. Just as you should never choose to undergo this surgery for someone else, you also should never feel as if you must rationalize your decision to others. If you are questioned by others about your decision, it's important to be open minded about the reasoning behind the questions.

Often, those contemplating surgery interpret others' inquiries about their decision as being filled with judgment when they are not. Many are quick to interpret these questions as hostile, when they are often driven more by curiosity. While there are certainly plenty of naturally thin people who believe that anyone suffering from obesity must be a contemptuous glutton, most Americans understand that the rules for weight gain and obesity are not fair. Rather than assuming that all questions about your surgery require a defensive stance, feel free to share your struggles with others and your hopes for what the surgery will do to improve your life. The war against obesity and weight loss surgery discrimination must be fought one opinion at a time and an open, honest approach to your decision and experiences is our best weapon against weight-based bias.

When a person who also suffers from obesity questions your decision, their curiosity may be driven by their own thoughts about the surgery. The decision to undergo weight loss surgery is often a multi-year process and the person asking the questions may only be six months behind you in their decision-making process. If you feel comfortable, be open and honest. This can be a very emotionally complex conversation with many layers of feelings.

If you are similar sized or smaller than the person you are having the discussion with, the implications of your decision are clear - if you need surgery then they do too. This fact can be quite unpleasant for some to face. If the conversation feels uncomfortable, don't immediately assume that their resistance comes from a judgment against you. It's much more likely that their negative emotions come from their feelings about their own weight problems. Be understanding and resist any instincts to engage in an argument. Remember, you are making this decision for you and not for others. As you start to lose weight after surgery, you can be sure that others are watching. You shouldn't be surprised when someone who you initially thought was judgmental about your decision approaches you with questions about your experience in their quest to learn more about how they can be more successful in their weight loss struggles.

Deciding who to tell about your decision is very personal and varies tremendously from person to person. Some people immediately announce their decision on Facebook and are quick to tell anyone who asks about their weight loss about their surgery. Others tell absolutely no one. I've even had a patient who didn't tell their spouse - I was instructed to explain that they were having surgery for their heartburn (it turned out that their spouse already knew and was just trying to respect the other's privacy). While I don't recommend this highly secretive approach, the decision about how to share your weight loss surgery experience is yours and yours alone to make.

Not everyone will agree with your choice, but this is to be expected. Some will be concerned for your safety, while others may offer resistance for reasons that are more about them than you. Others will support you wholeheartedly and wish you nothing but the best. It is likely you will have to deal with the entire spectrum of approval. Just remember, you are making this decision for you, not for them. Exploring the motivation behind a person's approval or disapproval will likely say more about who they are than about you and the decision that you are making.

CHAPTER THIRTEEN
FINAL THOUGHTS

Without question, Bariatric Surgery has been one of the most misunderstood fields of medicine over the past 30 years. For decades, we've been performing these surgeries and watching our patients' success without really understanding how and why these surgeries worked. As surgeons who are used to being listened to and respected, we've always thought that it was our serious tone of voice and powerful words of encouragement that finally allowed our patients to commit to lifestyle changes once and for all. Over the last decade, we've begun to recognize that psychological and emotional issues are likely secondary factors and it's the positive, fat burning hormonal state induced by Bariatric Surgery that is ultimately responsible for our patient's ability to finally lose weight and keep it off.

Now that we are beginning to understand the importance of the hormonal changes that result from our surgical interventions as the major force driving weight loss, we must also re-examine the recommendations we make to our patients. Recognizing surgery as a treatment that lowers the set point on our patient's metabolic thermostat demonstrates the importance of providing care for our patients that works to maximize and preserve this lowered set point.

Given this new perspective on success after surgery, our work must focus on maintaining the best environment to maintain this favorable hormonal state. This supports the importance of maintaining good nutrition after surgery- a high protein diet that emphasizes animal protein over fruit, vegetables, nuts, seeds and beans no longer makes sense. Additionally, choosing an exercise program that focuses on building muscle and strength over burning calories may be the wiser choice. Also, recognizing the potential set point raising effects of inactivity and injury, certain medications and processed foods like diet soda, sugar sweetened beverages and low-calorie junk food becomes a critically important component of your strategy for postoperative success.

We've all heard a patient describe his or her experience after weight loss surgery as a "journey." This new view of working to maximize the favorable hormonal balance and then maintain this new lowered set point emphasizes the wisdom of this perspective. Very few patients are lucky enough to reach their final goal weight and then easily maintain this new favorable body weight for the rest of their life. Many patients never achieve their ultimate weight loss goal and often battle weight regain in the years following their surgery. Although their struggles are now centered around a much lower weight, they are still struggling, nonetheless. These struggles are not a sign of personal failure, instead, they are temporary setbacks that will make you stronger in the end.

It is very likely that your journey will contain periods of smooth sailing as well as some time facing rough seas. To expect anything less from your postoperative experience is short-sighted and overly optimistic. There will be moments along the way that are cause for celebration and happiness, and there are likely to be difficult times as well. Looking at your struggles as a sign of personal failure ignores the courage and drive that has gotten you to this point. It is in these difficult moments that you will find the courage to re-examine your life choices and re-focus on the important things that have worked in the past and will work again in the future. Most bariatric programs offer services that can help to get you back on track, and the really good ones can work with you to identify factors outside of nutrition and exercise that may be contributing to your weight regain.

The key to your success and satisfaction lies both in establishing the most favorable environment to maximize your weight loss after surgery as well as recognizing that, like most other medical treatments, there are factors beyond your control that contribute to success and failure after weight loss surgery. Just as we emphasized in the early chapters that the weight that you gained in the years leading up to your surgery was not solely the result of a lack of willpower, we must now emphasize that the same logic continues to apply after surgery. There is a strong genetic component of your postoperative weight loss which lies squarely outside of your control.

While weight loss and health improvements after surgery are important, it is critical that you do not allow them to define you as a person. Your decision to undergo weight loss surgery was a calculated risk that you took that required great courage and any results that you achieve deserve to be celebrated. Remember, even the worst weight loss results after surgery would still be considered a tremendous success if they were achieved by any other mechanism.

Your weight loss is likely to attract attention which you may or may not welcome. It is critical that you remember that who you are is not reflected by the bathroom scale. The important people in your life who genuinely respect and care for you were not influenced by your weight before surgery and will be not be influenced afterward. Just as you were more than your weight before surgery, you are more than your weight loss afterward.

Many of you reading this have already had weight loss surgery and are looking for the keys to long term success. Others may be considering surgery or even planning on it. If you have already had surgery, I hope this book has provided a better understanding of the amazing opportunity that weight loss surgery can offer. If you are planning on surgery, I wish you a smooth recovery and a lifetime of weight loss success. But for all readers, I hope that this book has provided a better understanding of all of the causes and treatments of obesity and that this brings some peace to your struggles with your weight.

REFERENCES

[1] Nieuwdorp, Max, et al. "Role of the microbiome in energy regulation and metabolism." *Gastroenterology* 146.6 (2014): 1525-1533.

[2] Friedman, Jeffrey M., and Jeffrey L. Halaas. "Leptin and the regulation of body weight in mammals." *Nature* 395.6704 (1998): 763.

[3] Saper, Clifford B., Thomas C. Chou, and Joel K. Elmquist. "The need to feed: homeostatic and hedonic control of eating." *Neuron* 36.2 (2002): 199-211.

[4] Peach, MICHAEL J. "Renin-angiotensin system: biochemistry and mechanisms of action." *Physiological reviews* 57.2 (1977): 313-370.

[5] Folkow, Björn. "Nervous control of the blood vessels." *Physiological reviews* 35.3 (1955): 629-663.

[6] Von Euler, U. S. "Some aspects of the role of noradrenaline and adrenaline in circulation." *American heart journal* 56.3 (1958): 469-477.

[7] Prentice, Andrew, and Susan Jebb. "Energy intake/physical activity interactions in the homeostasis of body weight regulation." *Nutrition reviews* 62.suppl_2 (2004): S98-S104.

[8] Poehlman, Eric T., and Edward S. Horton. "The impact of food intake and exercise on energy expenditure." *Nutrition reviews*47.5 (1989): 129-137.

[9] Jéquier, Eric. "Energy expenditure in obesity." *Clinics in endocrinology and metabolism* 13.3 (1984): 563-580.

[10] Weigle, David S., et al. "Weight loss leads to a marked decrease in nonresting energy expenditure in ambulatory human subjects." *Metabolism* 37.10 (1988): 930-936.

[11] Silva, Analiza M., et al. "What is the effect of diet and/or exercise interventions on behavioural compensation in non-exercise physical activity and related energy expenditure of free-living adults? A systematic review." *British Journal of Nutrition* 119.12 (2018): 1327-1345.

[12] Schoffelen, P. F., and W. H. Saris. "Effects of addition of exercise to energy restriction on 24-hour energy expenditure, sleeping metabolic rate and daily physical activity." *European journal of clinical nutrition* 43.7 (1989): 441-451.

[13] Tremblay, Angela, et al. "Overfeeding and energy expenditure in humans." *The American journal of clinical nutrition* 56.5 (1992): 857-862.

[14] Roberts, SUSAN B., et al. "Energy expenditure and subsequent nutrient intakes in overfed young men." *American Journal of Physiology-Regulatory, Integrative and Comparative Physiology* 259.3 (1990): R461-R469.

[15] Franz, Marion J., et al. "Weight-loss outcomes: a systematic review and meta-analysis of weight-loss clinical trials with a minimum 1-year follow-up." *Journal of the American Dietetic Association* 107.10 (2007): 1755-1767.

[16] Arone, L. J., et al. "Autonomic nervous system activity in weight gain and weight

loss." *American Journal of Physiology-Regulatory, Integrative and Comparative Physiology* 269.1 (1995): R222-R225.

[17] Leibel, Rudolph L., Michael Rosenbaum, and Jules Hirsch. "Changes in energy expenditure resulting from altered body weight." *New England Journal of Medicine* 332.10 (1995): 621-628.

[18] Finkler, Elissa, Steven B. Heymsfield, and Marie-Pierre St-Onge. "Rate of weight loss can be predicted by patient characteristics and intervention strategies." *Journal of the Academy of Nutrition and Dietetics* 112.1 (2012): 75-80.

[19] Wyatt, Holly R., et al. "Resting energy expenditure in reduced-obese subjects in the National Weight Control Registry." *The American Journal of Clinical Nutrition* 69.6 (1999): 1189-1193.

[20] Pickering, Thomas G., et al. "Environmental influences on blood pressure and the role of job strain." *Journal of hypertension. Supplement: official journal of the International Society of Hypertension* 14.5 (1996): S179-85.

[21] Heller, Debra A., et al. "Genetic and environmental influences on serum lipid levels in twins." *New England Journal of Medicine* 328.16 (1993): 1150-1156.

[22] Ling, Charlotte, and Leif Groop. "Epigenetics: a molecular link between environmental factors and type 2 diabetes." *Diabetes*58.12 (2009): 2718-2725.

[23] AUSTIN, MELISSA A., et al. "Risk factors for coronary heart disease in adult female twins: genetic heritability and shared environmental influences." *American Journal of Epidemiology*125.2 (1987): 308-318.

[24] Verrotti, A., et al. "Weight gain following treatment with valproic acid: pathogenetic mechanisms and clinical implications." *obesity reviews* 12.5 (2011): e32-e43.

[25] Virkkunen, M., et al. "Decrease of energy expenditure causes weight increase in olanzapine treatment-a case study." *Pharmacopsychiatry* 35.03 (2002): 124-126.

[26] Clark, M. Kathleen, et al. "Weight, fat mass, and central distribution of fat increase when women use depot-medroxyprogesterone acetate for contraception." *International journal of Obesity* 29.10 (2005): 1252.

[27] Tataranni, PIETRO A., et al. "Effects of glucocorticoids on energy metabolism and food intake in humans." *American Journal of Physiology-Endocrinology and Metabolism* 271.2 (1996): E317-E325.

[28] Keck Jr, Paul E., and Susan L. McElroy. "Bipolar disorder, obesity, and pharmacotherapy-associated weight gain." *The Journal of clinical psychiatry* (2003).

[29] Semanscin-Doerr, Debra A., et al. "Mood disorders in laparoscopic sleeve gastrectomy patients: does it affect early weight loss?." *Surgery for Obesity and Related Diseases* 6.2 (2010): 191-196.

[30] Russell-Jones, David, and Rehman Khan. "Insulin-associated weight gain in diabetes–causes, effects and coping strategies." *Diabetes, Obesity and Metabolism* 9.6 (2007): 799-812.

[31] Weisler, Richard H., et al. "Comparison of bupropion and trazodone for the treatment of major depression." *Journal of clinical psychopharmacology* 14.3 (1994): 170-179.

[32] Safer, Daniel J. "A comparison of risperidone-induced weight gain across the age span." *Journal of clinical psychopharmacology* 24.4 (2004): 429-436.

[33] Fava, Maurizio. "Weight gain and antidepressants." *The Journal of clinical psychiatry* 61 (2000): 37-41.

[34] Carpenter, Sarah, and Lawrence S. Neinstein. "Weight gain in adolescent and young adult oral contraceptive users." *Journal of Adolescent Health Care* 7.5 (1986): 342-344.

[35] Pedersen, Bente K., and Mark A. Febbraio. "Muscles, exercise and obesity: skeletal muscle as a secretory organ." *Nature Reviews Endocrinology* 8.8 (2012): 457.

[36] Bandini, L. G., et al. "Energy expenditure during carbohydrate overfeeding in obese and nonobese adolescents." *American Journal of Physiology-Endocrinology and Metabolism* 256.3 (1989): E357-E367.

[37] Ifland, J. R., et al. "Refined food addiction: a classic substance use disorder." *Medical hypotheses* 72.5 (2009): 518-526.

[38] DiMeglio, Doreen P., and Richard D. Mattes. "Liquid versus solid carbohydrate: effects on food intake and body weight." *International journal of obesity* 24.6 (2000): 794.

[39] Mourao, D. M., et al. "Effects of food form on appetite and energy intake in lean and obese young adults." *International journal of obesity* 31.11 (2007): 1688.

[40] Rodin, Judith, et al. "Weight cycling and fat distribution." *International journal of obesity* 14.4 (1990): 303-310.

[41] Blair, Steven N., et al. "Body weight change, all-cause mortality, and cause-specific mortality in the Multiple Risk Factor Intervention Trial." *Annals of internal medicine* 119.7_Part_2 (1993): 749-757.

[42] Stöger, Reinhard. "The thrifty epigenotype: an acquired and heritable predisposition for obesity and diabetes?." *Bioessays* 30.2 (2008): 156-166.

[43] Hsu, LK George, et al. "Nonsurgical factors that influence the outcome of bariatric surgery: a review." *Psychosomatic medicine* 60.3 (1998): 338-346.

[44] Howie, G. J., et al. "Maternal nutritional history predicts obesity in adult offspring independent of postnatal diet." *The Journal of physiology* 587.4 (2009): 905-915.

[45] Maltais, M. L., J. Desroches, and I. J. Dionne. "Changes in muscle mass and strength after menopause." *J Musculoskelet Neuronal Interact* 9.4 (2009): 186-97.

[46] Kivimäki, Mika, et al. "Work stress, weight gain and weight loss: evidence for bidirectional effects of job strain on body mass index in the Whitehall II study." *International journal of obesity* 30.6 (2006): 982.

[47] Geliebter, Allan, et al. "Work-shift period and weight change." *Nutrition* 16.1 (2000): 27-29.

[48] Ebbeling, Cara B., et al. "A randomized trial of sugar-sweetened beverages and

adolescent body weight." *New England Journal of Medicine* 367.15 (2012): 1407-1416.

[49] Drenick, Ernst J., and Daisie Johnson. "Weight reduction by fasting and semistarvation in morbid obesity: long-term follow-up." *International journal of obesity* (1978).

[50] Mozaffarian, Dariush, et al. "Changes in diet and lifestyle and long-term weight gain in women and men." *New England Journal of Medicine* 364.25 (2011): 2392-2404.

[51] Hermsdorff, Helen Hermana M., et al. "A legume-based hypocaloric diet reduces proinflammatory status and improves metabolic features in overweight/obese subjects." *European journal of nutrition* 50.1 (2011): 61-69.

[52] Ledoux, T. A., Melanie D. Hingle, and Tom Baranowski. "Relationship of fruit and vegetable intake with adiposity: a systematic review." *Obesity reviews* 12.5 (2011): e143-e150.

[53] Tadross, J. A., and C. W. Le Roux. "The mechanisms of weight loss after bariatric surgery." *International journal of obesity* 33.S1 (2009): S28.

[54] Miras, Alexander D., and Carel W. le Roux. "Bariatric surgery and taste: novel mechanisms of weight loss." *Current opinion in gastroenterology* 26.2 (2010): 140-145.

[55] Shaw, Kelly A., et al. "Exercise for overweight or obesity." *Cochrane database of systematic reviews* 4 (2006).

[56] Wu, T., et al. "Long-term effectiveness of diet-plus-exercise interventions vs. diet-only interventions for weight loss: a meta-analysis." *Obesity reviews* 10.3 (2009): 313-323.

[57] Boström, Pontus, et al. "A PGC1-α-dependent myokine that drives brown-fat-like development of white fat and thermogenesis." *Nature* 481.7382 (2012): 463.

[58] Sedlock, DARLENE A., JEAN A. Fissinger, and CHRISTOPHER L. Melby. "Effect of exercise intensity and duration on postexercise energy expenditure." *Medicine and science in sports and exercise* 21.6 (1989): 662-666.

[59] Fry, Andrew C. "The role of resistance exercise intensity on muscle fibre adaptations." *Sports medicine* 34.10 (2004): 663-679.

[60] Alkahtani, Shaea A., et al. "Interval training intensity affects energy intake compensation in obese men." *International journal of sport nutrition and exercise metabolism* 24.6 (2014): 595-604.

[61] Hunter, G. R., et al. "A role for high intensity exercise on energy balance and weight control." *International journal of obesity* 22.6 (1998): 489.

[62] Anderson, N. B., et al. "Stress in America: Our health at risk." *Washington, DC: American Psychological Association* (2012).

[63] Irwin, Melinda L., et al. "Effect of exercise on total and intra-abdominal body fat in postmenopausal women: a randomized controlled trial." *Jama* 289.3 (2003): 323-330.

[64] Dombrowski, Stephan U., et al. "Long term maintenance of weight loss with non-surgical interventions in obese adults: systematic review and meta-analyses of randomised controlled trials." *Bmj* 348 (2014): g2646.

[65] Catenacci, Victoria A., et al. "Physical activity patterns in the national weight control registry." *Obesity* 16.1 (2008): 153-161.

[66] Catenacci, Victoria A., et al. "Physical activity patterns using accelerometry in the National Weight Control Registry." *Obesity* 19.6 (2011): 1163-1170.

[67] Fujioka, K., et al. "The relationship between early weight loss and weight loss at 1 year with naltrexone ER/bupropion ER combination therapy." *International Journal of Obesity* 40.9 (2016): 1369.

[68] Dhurandhar, N. V., et al. "Initial weight loss as a predictor of response to obesity drugs." *International journal of obesity* 23.12 (1999): 1333.

[69] Stanford, Fatima Cody, et al. "The utility of weight loss medications after bariatric surgery for weight regain or inadequate weight loss: a multi-center study." *Surgery for Obesity and Related Diseases* 13.3 (2017): 491-500.

[70] Silverstone, Trevor. "The anorectic effect of a long-acting preparation of phentermine (Duromine)." *Psychopharmacologia* 25.4 (1972): 315-320.

[71] Weintraub, Michael, et al. "Long-term weight control study V (weeks 190 to 210) Follow-up of participants after cessation of medication." *Clinical Pharmacology & Therapeutics* 51.5 (1992): 615-618.

[72] Bray, George A., et al. "A 6-month randomized, placebo-controlled, dose-ranging trial of topiramate for weight loss in obesity." *Obesity research* 11.6 (2003): 722-733.

[73] Shin, Jin Hee, and Kishore M. Gadde. "Clinical utility of phentermine/topiramate (Qsymia™) combination for the treatment of obesity." *Diabetes, metabolic syndrome and obesity: targets and therapy* 6 (2013): 131.

[74] Ornellas, Tehane, and Benjamin Chavez. "Naltrexone SR/Bupropion SR (Contrave): a new approach to weight loss in obese adults." *Pharmacy and Therapeutics* 36.5 (2011): 255.

[75] Gustafson, Ashley, Camille King, and Jose A. Rey. "Lorcaserin (Belviq): A selective serotonin 5-HT2C agonist in the treatment of obesity." *Pharmacy and Therapeutics* 38.9 (2013): 525.

[76] Vilsbøll, Tina, et al. "Effects of glucagon-like peptide-1 receptor agonists on weight loss: systematic review and meta-analyses of randomised controlled trials." *Bmj* 344 (2012): d7771.

[77] "Saxenda – Prices, Savings and Coupon Tips - GoodRx." Prescription Prices, Coupons & Pharmacy Information – *GoodRx*", GoodRX, 10/07/2019, https://www.goodrx.com/saxenda.

[78] Xia, Ying, et al. "Treatment of obesity: Pharmacotherapy trends in the U nited S tates from 1999 to 2010." *Obesity* 23.8 (2015): 1721-1728.

[79] le Roux, Carel W., et al. "Gut hormones as mediators of appetite and weight loss after Roux-en-Y gastric bypass." *Annals of surgery* 246.5 (2007): 780-785.

[80] le Roux, Carel W., et al. "Gut hormone profiles following bariatric surgery favor an anorectic state, facilitate weight loss, and improve metabolic parameters." *Annals of*

surgery 243.1 (2006): 108.

[81] Cummings, David E., et al. "Plasma ghrelin levels after diet-induced weight loss or gastric bypass surgery." *New England Journal of Medicine* 346.21 (2002): 1623-1630.

[82] Tam, C. S., et al. "Could the mechanisms of bariatric surgery hold the key for novel therapies?: report from a Pennington Scientific Symposium." *Obesity reviews* 12.11 (2011): 984-994.

[83] Cushing, Christopher C., et al. "Longitudinal trends in food cravings following Roux-en-Y gastric bypass in an adolescent sample." *Surgery for Obesity and Related Diseases* 11.1 (2015): 14-18.

[84] Stylopoulos, Nicholas, Alison G. Hoppin, and Lee M. Kaplan. "Roux-en-Y gastric bypass enhances energy expenditure and extends lifespan in diet-induced obese rats." *Obesity* 17.10 (2009): 1839-1847.

[85] Abdeen, G., and C. W. Le Roux. "Mechanism underlying the weight loss and complications of Roux-en-Y gastric bypass. Review." *Obesity surgery* 26.2 (2016): 410-421.

[86] Cooper, Timothy C., et al. "Trends in weight regain following Roux-en-Y gastric bypass (RYGB) bariatric surgery." *Obesity surgery* 25.8 (2015): 1474-1481.

[87] Charidemou, Evelina, et al. "A randomized 3-way crossover study indicates that high-protein feeding induces de novo lipogenesis in healthy humans." *J Al-Najim, Werd, Neil G. Docherty, and Carel W. le Roux. "Food intake and eating behavior after bariatric surgery." Physiological reviews 98.3 (2018): 1113-1141. CI insight* 4.12 (2019).

[88] Al-Najim, Werd, Neil G. Docherty, and Carel W. le Roux. "Food intake and eating behavior after bariatric surgery." *Physiological reviews* 98.3 (2018): 1113-1141.

[89] Kassirer, Jerome P., and Marcia Angell. "Losing weight—an ill-fated New Year's resolution." (1998): 52-54.

[90] Garner, David M., and Susan C. Wooley. "Confronting the failure of behavioral and dietary treatments for obesity." *Clinical Psychology Review* 11.6 (1991): 729-780.

[91] Dey, Debashish Kumar, et al. "Height and body weight in the elderly. I. A 25-year longitudinal study of a population aged 70 to 95 years." *European Journal of Clinical Nutrition* 53.12 (1999): 905.

[92] Stein, Patricia M., Ruth S. Hassanein, and Barbara P. Lukert. "Predicting weight loss success among obese clients in a hospital nutrition clinic." *The American journal of clinical nutrition* 34.10 (1981): 2039-2044.

[93] Saris, Wim HM. "Very-low-calorie diets and sustained weight loss." *Obesity research* 9.S11 (2001): 295S-301S.

[94] Zamboni, Mauro, et al. "Sarcopenic obesity: a new category of obesity in the elderly." *Nutrition, Metabolism and Cardiovascular Diseases* 18.5 (2008): 388-395.

[95] Finks, Jonathan F., et al. "Predicting risk for serious complications with bariatric surgery: results from the Michigan Bariatric Surgery Collaborative." *Annals of surgery* 254.4 (2011):

633-640.

[96] Moreno-Aliaga, M. J., et al. "Does weight loss prognosis depend on genetic make-up?." *Obesity reviews* 6.2 (2005): 155-168.

[97] Loos, Ruth JF. "Genetic determinants of common obesity and their value in prediction." *Best practice & research Clinical endocrinology & metabolism* 26.2 (2012): 211-226.

[98] Hatoum, Ida J., et al. "Heritability of the weight loss response to gastric bypass surgery." *The Journal of Clinical Endocrinology & Metabolism* 96.10 (2011): E1630-E1633.

[99] Benoit, Stephen C., et al. "Use of bariatric outcomes longitudinal database (BOLD) to study variability in patient success after bariatric surgery." *Obesity surgery* 24.6 (2014): 936-943.

[100] El-Hayek, K., et al. "Marginal ulcer after Roux-en-Y gastric bypass: what have we really learned?." *Surgical endoscopy* 26.10 (2012): 2789-2796.

[101] Fox, S. Ross, et al. "The Lap-Band® system in a North American population." *Obesity surgery* 13.2 (2003): 275-280.

[102] O'brien, Paul E., et al. "Systematic review of medium-term weight loss after bariatric operations." *Obesity surgery* 16.8 (2006): 1032-1040.

[103] O'Brien, Paul E., and John B. Dixon. "Lap-Band®: outcomes and results." *Journal of Laparoendoscopic & Advanced Surgical Techniques* 13.4 (2003): 265-270.

[104] Korner, Judith, et al. "Prospective study of gut hormone and metabolic changes after adjustable gastric banding and Roux-en-Y gastric bypass." *International journal of obesity* 33.7 (2009): 786.

[105] Tsai, Catherine, et al. "Long-term outcomes and frequency of reoperative bariatric surgery beyond 15 years after gastric banding: a high band failure rate with safe revisions." *Surgery for Obesity and Related Diseases* (2019).

[106] Dargent, Jerome. "Laparoscopic gastric banding: game over?." *Obesity surgery* 27.8 (2017): 1914-1916.

[107] Lazzati, Andrea, et al. "Natural history of adjustable gastric banding: lifespan and revisional rate." *Annals of surgery* 265.3 (2017): 439-445.

[108] Prachand, Vivek N., Roy T. DaVee, and John C. Alverdy. "Duodenal switch provides superior weight loss in the super-obese (BMI≥ 50kg/m2) compared with gastric bypass." *Annals of surgery* 244.4 (2006): 611.

[109] Löfling Skogar, Martin, and Magnus Sundbom. "Risk of perioperative complications and adverse events the First Ten Years after Duodenal Switch and Gastric Bypass in a Matched National Cohort." (2019).

[110] Parikh, Manish S., et al. "Objective comparison of complications resulting from laparoscopic bariatric procedures." *Journal of the American College of Surgeons* 202.2 (2006): 252-261.

[111] Parrott, Julie, et al. "American Society for Metabolic and Bariatric Surgery integrated health nutritional guidelines for the surgical weight loss patient 2016 update: micronutrients." *Surgery for Obesity and Related Diseases* 13.5 (2017): 727-741.

[112] Buchwald, Henry, et al. "Weight and type 2 diabetes after bariatric surgery: systematic review and meta-analysis." *The American journal of medicine* 122.3 (2009): 248-256.

[113] Søvik, Torgeir T., et al. "Gastrointestinal function and eating behavior after gastric bypass and duodenal switch." *Surgery for Obesity and Related Diseases* 9.5 (2013): 641-647.

[114] Mason, EDWARD E., and Chikashi Ito. "Gastric bypass." *Annals of surgery* 170.3 (1969): 329.

[115] Griffen Jr, WARD O., V. LEROY Young, and CRAIG C. Stevenson. "A prospective comparison of gastric and jejunoileal bypass procedures for morbid obesity." *Annals of surgery* 186.4 (1977): 500.

[116] Sugerman, HARVEY J., JANET V. Starkey, and R. E. G. I. N. E. Birkenhauer. "A randomized prospective trial of gastric bypass versus vertical banded gastroplasty for morbid obesity and their effects on sweets versus non-sweets eaters." *Annals of surgery* 205.6 (1987): 613.

[117] Scopinaro, Nicola, et al. "Bilio-pancreatic bypass for obesity: II. Initial experience in man." *British Journal of Surgery* 66.9 (1979): 618-620.

[118] Angrisani, Luigi, Michele Lorenzo, and Vincenzo Borrelli. "Laparoscopic adjustable gastric banding versus Roux-en-Y gastric bypass: 5-year results of a prospective randomized trial." *Surgery for obesity and related diseases* 3.2 (2007): 127-132.

[119] Ignat, M., et al. "Randomized trial of Roux-en-Y gastric bypass versus sleeve gastrectomy in achieving excess weight loss." *British Journal of Surgery* 104.3 (2017): 248-256.

[120] American Society for Metabolic and Bariatric Surgery. (2019). *Estimate of Bariatric Surgery Numbers, 2011-2017 | American Society for Metabolic and Bariatric Surgery*. [online] Available at: https://asmbs.org/resources/estimate-of-bariatric-surgery-numbers [Accessed 21 Jul. 2019].

[121] Lynn, W., et al. "Laparoscopic Roux-en-Y gastric bypass is as safe as laparoscopic sleeve gastrectomy. Results of a comparative cohort study." *Annals of medicine and surgery* 35 (2018): 38-43.

[122] Ahmed, Bestoun, et al. "Long-term weight change and health outcomes for sleeve gastrectomy (SG) and matched Roux-en-Y gastric bypass (RYGB) participants in the Longitudinal Assessment of Bariatric Surgery (LABS) study." *Surgery* 164.4 (2018): 774-783.

[123] Carlin, Arthur M., et al. "The comparative effectiveness of sleeve gastrectomy, gastric bypass, and adjustable gastric banding procedures for the treatment of morbid obesity." *Annals of surgery* 257.5 (2013): 791-797.

[124] Shoar, Saeed, and Alan A. Saber. "Long-term and midterm outcomes of laparoscopic

sleeve gastrectomy versus Roux-en-Y gastric bypass: a systematic review and meta-analysis of comparative studies." *Surgery for Obesity and Related Diseases* 13.2 (2017): 170-180.

[125] Kruljac, Ivan, et al. "Changes in metabolic hormones after bariatric surgery and their predictive impact on weight loss." *Clinical endocrinology* 85.6 (2016): 852-860.

[126] Holsen, Laura M., et al. "Neural predictors of 12-month weight loss outcomes following bariatric surgery." *International Journal of Obesity* 42.4 (2018): 785.

[127] Dirksen, C., et al. "Gut hormones, early dumping and resting energy expenditure in patients with good and poor weight loss response after Roux-en-Y gastric bypass." *International journal of obesity* 37.11 (2013): 1452.

[128] Alamuddin, Naji, et al. "Changes in fasting and prandial gut and adiposity hormones following vertical sleeve gastrectomy or Roux-en-Y-gastric bypass: an 18-month prospective study." *Obesity surgery* 27.6 (2017): 1563-1572.

[129] Adil, Md Tanveer, et al. "A Systematic Review and Meta-Analysis of the Effect of Roux-en-Y Gastric Bypass on Barrett's Esophagus." *Obesity surgery* (2019): 1-10.

[130] Santonicola, Antonella, et al. "Hiatal hernia diagnosis prospectively assessed in obese patients before bariatric surgery: accuracy of high-resolution manometry taking intraoperative diagnosis as reference standard." *Surgical endoscopy* (2019): 1-7.

[131] Samakar, Kamran, et al. "The effect of laparoscopic sleeve gastrectomy with concomitant hiatal hernia repair on gastroesophageal reflux disease in the morbidly obese." *Obesity surgery* 26.1 (2016): 61-66.

[132] Docimo, Salvatore, et al. "Concomitant hiatal hernia repair is more common in laparoscopic sleeve gastrectomy than during laparoscopic Roux-en-Y Gastric bypass: an analysis of 130,772 cases." *Obesity surgery* 29.2 (2019): 744-746.

[133] Nilsson, M., et al. "Lifestyle related risk factors in the aetiology of gastro-oesophageal reflux." *Gut* 53.12 (2004): 1730-1735.

[134] Carter, Patrice R., et al. "Association between gastroesophageal reflux disease and laparoscopic sleeve gastrectomy." *Surgery for obesity and related diseases* 7.5 (2011): 569-572

[135] Pories, Walter J., et al. "The control of diabetes mellitus (NIDDM) in the morbidly obese with the Greenville Gastric Bypass." *Annals of surgery* 206.3 (1987): 316.

[136] Brethauer, Stacy A., et al. "Can diabetes be surgically cured?: long-term metabolic effects of bariatric surgery in obese patients with type 2 diabetes mellitus." *Annals of surgery* 258.4 (2013): 628.

[137] Li, Jian-Fang, et al. "Comparison of laparoscopic Roux-en-Y gastric bypass with laparoscopic sleeve gastrectomy for morbid obesity or type 2 diabetes mellitus: a meta-analysis of randomized controlled trials." *Canadian Journal of Surgery* 56.6 (2013): E158.

[138] Lee, Wei-Jei, et al. "Gastric bypass vs sleeve gastrectomy for type 2 diabetes mellitus: a randomized controlled trial." *Archives of surgery* 146.2 (2011): 143-148.

[139] American Society for Metabolic and Bariatric Surgery. (2012). Studies Weigh in on Safety

and Effectiveness of Newer Bariatric and Metabolic Surgery Procedure | American Society for Metabolic and Bariatric Surgery. [online] Available at: https://asmbs.org/resources/studies-weigh-in-on-safety-and-effectiveness-of-newer-bariatric-and-metabolic-surgery-procedure [Accessed 27 Jul. 2019].

[140] Gribsholt, Sigrid Bjerge, et al. "Rate of acute hospital admissions before and after roux-en-y gastric bypass surgery." *Annals of surgery* 267.2 (2018): 319-325.

[141] Pontiroli, Antonio E., and Alberto Morabito. "Long-term prevention of mortality in morbid obesity through bariatric surgery. a systematic review and meta-analysis of trials performed with gastric banding and gastric bypass." Annals of surgery 253.3 (2011): 484-487.

[142] Adams, Ted D., et al. "Long-term mortality after gastric bypass surgery." New England Journal of Medicine 357.8 (2007): 753-761.

[143] Obeid, Nabeel R., et al. "Long-term outcomes after Roux-en-Y gastric bypass: 10-to 13-year data." Surgery for Obesity and Related Diseases 12.1 (2016): 11-20.

[144] Bruze, Gustaf, et al. "Hospital admission after gastric bypass: a nationwide cohort study with up to 6 years follow-up." Surgery for Obesity and Related Diseases 13.6 (2017): 962-969.

[145] Brolin, R. E., et al. "Are vitamin B 12 and folate deficiency clinically important after Roux-en-Y gastric bypass?." Journal of Gastrointestinal Surgery 2.5 (1998): 436-442.

[146] Karefylakis, Christos, et al. "Prevalence of anemia and related deficiencies 10 years after gastric bypass—a retrospective study." Obesity surgery 25.6 (2015): 1019-1023.

[147] Sahebzamani, Frances M., Adrienne Berarducci, and Michel M. Murr. "Malabsorption anemia and iron supplement induced constipation in post-Roux-en-Y gastric bypass (RYGB) patients." Journal of the American Association of Nurse Practitioners 25.12 (2013): 634-640.

[148] Kotkiewicz, Adam, et al. "Anemia and the need for intravenous iron infusion after Roux-en-Y gastric bypass." Clinical Medicine Insights: Blood Disorders 8 (2015): CMBD-S21825.

[149] Parrott, Julie, et al. "American Society for Metabolic and Bariatric Surgery integrated health nutritional guidelines for the surgical weight loss patient 2016 update: micronutrients." Surgery for Obesity and Related Diseases 13.5 (2017): 727-741.

[150] Ahmed, Ahmed R., et al. "Trends in internal hernia incidence after laparoscopic Roux-en-Y gastric bypass." Obesity surgery17.12 (2007): 1563-1566.

[151] Higa, Kelvin D., Tienchin Ho, and Keith B. Boone. "Internal hernias after laparoscopic Roux-en-Y gastric bypass: incidence, treatment and prevention." Obesity Surgery 13.3 (2003): 350-354.

[152] Parakh, Shwetambara, Eliana Soto, and Stephen Merola. "Diagnosis and management of internal hernias after laparoscopic gastric bypass." Obesity surgery 17.11 (2007): 1498-1502.

[153] Coblijn, Usha K., et al. "Development of ulcer disease after Roux-en-Y gastric bypass,

incidence, risk factors, and patient presentation: a systematic review." *Obesity surgery* 24.2 (2014): 299-309.

[154] Azagury, D. E., et al. "Marginal ulceration after Roux-en-Y gastric bypass surgery: characteristics, risk factors, treatment, and outcomes." *Endoscopy* 43.11 (2011): 950-954.

[155] Mulle, Jennifer G., William G. Sharp, and Joseph F. Cubells. "The gut microbiome: a new frontier in autism research." *Current psychiatry reports* 15.2 (2013): 337.

[156] Jangi, Sushrut, et al. "Alterations of the human gut microbiome in multiple sclerosis." *Nature communications* 7 (2016): 12015.

[157] Gevers, Dirk, et al. "The treatment-naive microbiome in new-onset Crohn's disease." *Cell host & microbe* 15.3 (2014): 382-392.

[158] Turnbaugh, Peter J., et al. "An obesity-associated gut microbiome with increased capacity for energy harvest." *nature* 444.7122 (2006): 1027.

[159] Chen, Jung-Chien, et al. "Effect of probiotics on postoperative quality of gastric bypass surgeries: a prospective randomized trial." *Surgery for Obesity and Related Diseases* 12.1 (2016): 57-61.

[160] Li, Vicky Ka Ming, et al. "Predictors of gallstone formation after bariatric surgery: a multivariate analysis of risk factors comparing gastric bypass, gastric banding, and sleeve gastrectomy." *Surgical endoscopy* 23.7 (2009): 1640-1644.

[161] Wood, Bernard, and Alison Brooks. "Human evolution: We are what we ate." *Nature* 400.6741 (1999): 219.

[162] Hessler, Paul C., et al. "High accuracy sonographic recognition of gallstones." *American Journal of Roentgenology* 136.3 (1981): 517-520.

[163] Wanjura, Viktor, et al. "Cholecystectomy after gastric bypass—incidence and complications." *Surgery for Obesity and Related Diseases* 13.6 (2017): 979-987.

[164] Ceppa, Federico A., et al. "Laparoscopic transgastric endoscopy after Roux-en-Y gastric bypass." *Surgery for Obesity and Related Diseases* 3.1 (2007): 21-24.

[165] Villegas, Leonardo, et al. "Is routine cholecystectomy required during laparoscopic gastric bypass?." *Obesity surgery* 14.2 (2004): 206-211.

[166] Li, Linlin, and Li-Tzy Wu. "Substance use after bariatric surgery: A review." *Journal of psychiatric research* 76 (2016): 16-29.

[167] Klockhoff, H., I. Näslund, and A. Wayne Jones. "Faster absorption of ethanol and higher peak concentration in women after gastric bypass surgery." *British journal of clinical pharmacology* 54.6 (2002): 587-591.

[168] Svensson, Per-Arne, et al. "Alcohol consumption and alcohol problems after bariatric surgery in the Swedish obese subjects study." *Obesity* 21.12 (2013): 2444-2451.

[169] Woodard, Gavitt A., et al. "Impaired alcohol metabolism after gastric bypass surgery: a case-crossover trial." *Journal of the American College of Surgeons* 212.2 (2011): 209-214.

[170] Parikh, Manish, Jason M. Johnson, and Naveen Ballem. "ASMBS position statement on

alcohol use before and after bariatric surgery." *Surgery for Obesity and Related Diseases*12.2 (2016): 225-230.

[171] Deitel, Mervyn, Ross D. Crosby, and Michel Gagner. "The first international consensus summit for sleeve gastrectomy (SG), New York City, October 25–27, 2007." *Obesity surgery* 18.5 (2008): 487-496.

[172] Dimitriadis, Efstathios, et al. "Alterations in gut hormones after laparoscopic sleeve gastrectomy: a prospective clinical and laboratory investigational study." *Annals of surgery* 257.4 (2013): 647-654.

[173] Peterli, Ralph, et al. "Metabolic and hormonal changes after laparoscopic Roux-en-Y gastric bypass and sleeve gastrectomy: a randomized, prospective trial." *Obesity surgery*22.5 (2012): 740-748.

[174] Thereaux, Jérémie, et al. "Comparison of results after one year between sleeve gastrectomy and gastric bypass in patients with BMI≥ 50 kg/m². " *Surgery for Obesity and Related Diseases* 11.4 (2015): 785-790.

[175] Makaronidis, Janine M., et al. "Reported appetite, taste and smell changes following Roux-en-Y gastric bypass and sleeve gastrectomy: effect of gender, type 2 diabetes and relationship to post-operative weight loss." *Appetite* 107 (2016): 93-105.

[176] Rrezza, E. E., et al. "Symptomatic improvement in gastroesophageal reflux disease (GERD) following laparoscopic Roux-en-Y gastric bypass." *Surgical endoscopy*16.7 (2002): 1027-1031.

[177] Samakar, Kamran, et al. "The effect of laparoscopic sleeve gastrectomy with concomitant hiatal hernia repair on gastroesophageal reflux disease in the morbidly obese." *Obesity surgery* 26.1 (2016): 61-66.

[178] Felsenreich, Daniel M., et al. "Weight loss, weight regain, and conversions to Roux-en-Y gastric bypass: 10-year results of laparoscopic sleeve gastrectomy." *Surgery for Obesity and Related Diseases* 12.9 (2016): 1655-1662.

[179] Mandeville, Yannick, et al. "Moderating the enthusiasm of sleeve gastrectomy: up to fifty percent of reflux symptoms after ten years in a consecutive series of one hundred laparoscopic sleeve gastrectomies." *Obesity surgery* 27.7 (2017): 1797-1803.

[180] Varban, Oliver A., et al. "Surgeon variation in severity of reflux symptoms after sleeve gastrectomy." *Surgical Endoscopy*(2019): 1-7.

[181] Peterli, Ralph, et al. "Effect of laparoscopic sleeve gastrectomy vs laparoscopic Roux-en-Y gastric bypass on weight loss in patients with morbid obesity: the SM-BOSS randomized clinical trial." *Jama* 319.3 (2018): 255-265.

[182] Parmar, Chetan D., et al. "Conversion of sleeve gastrectomy to Roux-en-Y gastric bypass is effective for gastro-oesophageal reflux disease but not for further weight loss." *Obesity surgery* 27.7 (2017): 1651-1658.

[183] Genco, Alfredo, et al. "Gastroesophageal reflux disease and Barrett's esophagus after laparoscopic sleeve gastrectomy: a possible, underestimated long-term

complication." *Surgery for Obesity and Related Diseases* 13.4 (2017): 568-574.

[184] Hvid-Jensen, Frederik, et al. "Incidence of adenocarcinoma among patients with Barrett's esophagus." *New England Journal of Medicine* 365.15 (2011): 1375-1383.

[185] Khidir, Nesreen, et al. "Initial experience of endoscopic radiofrequency waves delivery to the lower esophageal sphincter (Stretta procedure) on symptomatic gastroesophageal reflux disease post-sleeve gastrectomy." *Obesity surgery* 28.10 (2018): 3125-3130.

[186] Vilallonga, Ramon, Jacques Himpens, and Simon van de Vrande. "Laparoscopic management of persistent strictures after laparoscopic sleeve gastrectomy." *Obesity surgery* 23.10 (2013): 1655-1661.

[187] Hawasli, Abdelkader, et al. "Laparoscopic placement of the LINX® system in management of severe reflux after sleeve gastrectomy." *The American Journal of Surgery* 217.3 (2019): 496-499.

[188] Soong, Tien-Chou, et al. "Revision of Sleeve Gastrectomy with Hiatal Repair with Gastropexy for Gastroesophageal Reflux Disease." *Obesity surgery* (2019): 1-6.

[189] Adams, Lindsay B., et al. "Randomized, prospective comparison of ursodeoxycholic acid for the prevention of gallstones after sleeve gastrectomy." *Obesity surgery* 26.5 (2016): 990-994.

[190] Warschkow, Rene, et al. "Concomitant cholecystectomy during laparoscopic Roux-en-Y gastric bypass in obese patients is not justified: a meta-analysis." *Obesity surgery* 23.3 (2013): 397-407.

[191] Hessler, Paul C., et al. "High accuracy sonographic recognition of gallstones." *American Journal of Roentgenology* 136.3 (1981): 517-520.

[192] Sakran, Nasser, et al. "Laparoscopic sleeve gastrectomy for morbid obesity in 3003 patients: results at a high-volume bariatric center." *Obesity surgery* 26.9 (2016): 2045-2050.

[193] Al-Sabah, Salman, Martin Ladouceur, and Nicolas Christou. "Anastomotic leaks after bariatric surgery: it is the host response that matters." *Surgery for Obesity and Related Diseases* 4.2 (2008): 152-157.

[194] Yehoshua, Ronit T., et al. "Laparoscopic sleeve gastrectomy—volume and pressure assessment." *Obesity surgery* 18.9 (2008): 1083.

[195] Sakran, Nasser, et al. "Gastric leaks after sleeve gastrectomy: a multicenter experience with 2,834 patients." *Surgical endoscopy* 27.1 (2013): 240-245.

[196] Aminian, A., et al. "How safe is metabolic/diabetes surgery?." *Diabetes, Obesity and Metabolism* 17.2 (2015): 198-201.

[197] Sjöström, Lars, et al. "Effects of bariatric surgery on mortality in Swedish obese subjects." *New England journal of medicine* 357.8 (2007): 741-752.

[198] Christou, Nicolas V., et al. "Surgery decreases long-term mortality, morbidity, and health care use in morbidly obese patients." *Annals of surgery* 240.3 (2004): 416.

[199] Schauer, Daniel P., et al. "Impact of bariatric surgery on life expectancy in severely obese patients with diabetes: a decision analysis." *Annals of surgery* 261.5 (2015): 914.

[200] Chang, William W., et al. "Factors influencing long-term weight loss after bariatric surgery." *Surgery for Obesity and Related Diseases* 15.3 (2019): 456-461.

[201] Hanvold, Susanna E., et al. "Does Lifestyle Intervention After Gastric Bypass Surgery Prevent Weight Regain? A Randomized Clinical Trial." *Obesity surgery* (2019): 1-13.

[202] Kafri, Naama, et al. "Health behavior, food tolerance, and satisfaction after laparoscopic sleeve gastrectomy." *Surgery for Obesity and Related Diseases* 7.1 (2011): 82-88.

[203] Gjessing, Hanne Rosendahl, et al. "Energy intake, nutritional status and weight reduction in patients one year after laparoscopic sleeve gastrectomy." *SpringerPlus* 2.1 (2013): 352.

[204] Colles, Susan L., John B. Dixon, and Paul E. O'brien. "Grazing and loss of control related to eating: two high-risk factors following bariatric surgery." *Obesity* 16.3 (2008): 615-622.

[205] Coluzzi, Ilenia, et al. "Food intake and changes in eating behavior after laparoscopic sleeve gastrectomy." *Obesity surgery* 26.9 (2016): 2059-2067.

[206] Ramadan, M., et al. "Risk of dumping syndrome after sleeve gastrectomy and Roux-en-Y gastric bypass: early results of a multicentre prospective study." *Gastroenterology research and practice* 2016 (2016).

[207] Altieri, Maria S., et al. "Rate of revisions or conversion after bariatric surgery over 10 years in the state of New York." *Surgery for Obesity and Related Diseases* 14.4 (2018): 500-507.

[208] Janik, Michal R., et al. "Safety of revision sleeve gastrectomy compared to Roux-Y gastric bypass after failed gastric banding: analysis of the MBSAQIP." *Annals of surgery* 269.2 (2019): 299-303.

[209] Wu, Chang, et al. "Clinical Outcomes of Sleeve Gastrectomy Versus Roux-En-Y Gastric Bypass After Failed Adjustable Gastric Banding." *Obesity surgery* (2019): 1-12.

[210] Chowbey, Pradeep K., et al. "Laparoscopic Roux-en-Y gastric bypass: outcomes of a case-matched comparison of primary versus revisional surgery." *Journal of minimal access surgery* 14.1 (2018): 52.

[211] Goldberg, Michael, et al. "Laparoscopic Limb Distalization for Failed Roux-en-Y Gastric Bypass." *Surgery for Obesity and Related Diseases* 13.10 (2017): S169.

[212] Felsenreich, Daniel M., et al. "Surgical Therapy of Weight Regain Following Roux-en-Y Gastric Bypass." *Surgery for Obesity and Related Diseases* (2019).

[213] Gallo, Alberto S., et al. "Endoscopic revision of gastric bypass: Holy Grail or Epic fail?." *Surgical endoscopy* 30.9 (2016): 3922-3927.

[214] Nevo, Nadav, et al. "Converting a sleeve gastrectomy to a gastric bypass for weight loss failure—is it worth it?." *Obesity surgery* 28.2 (2018): 364-368.

[215] Carmeli, Idan, et al. "Laparoscopic conversion of sleeve gastrectomy to a biliopancreatic

diversion with duodenal switch or a Roux-en-Y gastric bypass due to weight loss failure: our algorithm." *Surgery for Obesity and Related Diseases* 11.1 (2015): 79-85.

[216] Kim, Julie. "American Society for Metabolic and Bariatric Surgery statement on single-anastomosis duodenal switch." *Surgery for Obesity and Related Diseases* 12.5 (2016): 944-945.

[217] Poghosyan, Tigran, et al. "Conversion of Sleeve Gastrectomy to One Anastomosis Gastric Bypass for Weight Loss Failure." *Obesity surgery* (2019): 1-6.

[218] Varban, Oliver A., et al. "Analysis of Self vs Peer Ratings of Surgical Skill with Bariatric Surgery." *Surgery for Obesity and Related Diseases* 14.11 (2018): S70.

[219] Ju, Tammy, et al. "Barriers to bariatric surgery: Factors influencing progression to bariatric surgery in a US metropolitan area." *Surgery for Obesity and Related Diseases* 15.2 (2019): 261-268.

[220] Keith Jr, Charles J., et al. "Insurance-mandated preoperative diet and outcomes after bariatric surgery." *Surgery for Obesity and Related Diseases* 14.5 (2018): 631-636.

[221] Pearl, Rebecca L., et al. "Reconsidering the Psychosocial-Behavioral Evaluation Required Prior to Bariatric Surgery." *Obesity* 26.2 (2018): 249-250.

[222] Weiner, Matthew. *A Pound of Cure: Change Your Eating and Your Life, One Step at a Time*. Createspace, 2013.

[223] Leenders, Max, et al. "Fruit and vegetable consumption and mortality: European prospective investigation into cancer and nutrition." *American journal of epidemiology* 178.4 (2013): 590-602.

[224] Fuhrman, Joel. *Nutritarian Handbook and ANDI Food Scoring Guide*. Gift of Health Press, 2012.

[225] Rolls, Barbara J., Julia A. Ello-Martin, and Beth Carlton Tohill. "What can intervention studies tell us about the relationship between fruit and vegetable consumption and weight management?." *Nutrition reviews* 62.1 (2004): 1-17.

[226] Speth, John D. "Early hominid hunting and scavenging: the role of meat as an energy source." *Journal of Human Evolution* 18.4 (1989): 329-343.

[227] Barker, Lewis M. *The psychobiology of human food selection*. AVI Pub. Co., 1982.

[228] Mozaffarian, Dariush, et al. "Changes in diet and lifestyle and long-term weight gain in women and men." *New England Journal of Medicine* 364.25 (2011): 2392-2404.

[229] He, Ka, et al. "Changes in intake of fruits and vegetables in relation to risk of obesity and weight gain among middle-aged women." *International journal of obesity* 28.12 (2004): 1569.

[230] Bes-Rastrollo, Maira, et al. "Association of fiber intake and fruit/vegetable consumption with weight gain in a Mediterranean population." *Nutrition* 22.5 (2006): 504-511.

[231] DellaValle, Diane M., Liane S. Roe, and Barbara J. Rolls. "Does the consumption of caloric and non-caloric beverages with a meal affect energy intake?." *Appetite* 44.2 (2005):

187-193.

[232] Almiron-Roig, Eva, and Adam Drewnowski. "Hunger, thirst, and energy intakes following consumption of caloric beverages." *Physiology & behavior* 79.4-5 (2003): 767-773.

[233] Saris, Wim HM. "Sugars, energy metabolism, and body weight control." *The American journal of clinical nutrition* 78.4 (2003): 850S-857S.

[234] Schulze, Matthias B., et al. "Sugar-sweetened beverages, weight gain, and incidence of type 2 diabetes in young and middle-aged women." *Jama* 292.8 (2004): 927-934.

[235] Popkin, Barry M., and Samara Joy Nielsen. "The sweetening of the world's diet." *Obesity research* 11.11 (2003): 1325-1332.

[236] Olsen, N. J., and B. L. Heitmann. "Intake of calorically sweetened beverages and obesity." *Obesity reviews* 10.1 (2009): 68-75.

[237] Tordoff, Michael G., and Annette M. Alleva. "Effect of drinking soda sweetened with aspartame or high-fructose corn syrup on food intake and body weight." *The American journal of clinical nutrition* 51.6 (1990): 963-969.

[238] de La Peña, Carolyn. "Artificial sweetener as a historical window to culturally situated health." *Annals of the New York Academy of Sciences* 1190.1 (2010): 159-165.

[239] Fowler, Sharon P., et al. "Fueling the obesity epidemic? Artificially sweetened beverage use and long-term weight gain." *Obesity* 16.8 (2008): 1894-1900.

[240] Fowler, Sharon P., et al. "Fueling the obesity epidemic? Artificially sweetened beverage use and long-term weight gain." *Obesity* 16.8 (2008): 1894-1900.

[241] Mcburney, Donald H. "Gustatory cross adaptation between sweet-tasting compounds." *Perception & Psychophysics* 11.3 (1972): 225-227.

[242] Appleton, K. M., and J. E. Blundell. "Habitual high and low consumers of artificially-sweetened beverages: effects of sweet taste and energy on short-term appetite." *Physiology & behavior* 92.3 (2007): 479-486.

243 Burke, Mary V., and Dana M. Small. "Physiological mechanisms by which non-nutritive sweeteners may impact body weight and metabolism." Physiology & behavior 152 (2015): 381-388.

244 Swithers, Susan E. "Artificial sweeteners produce the counterintuitive effect of inducing metabolic derangements." *Trends in Endocrinology & Metabolism* 24.9 (2013): 431-441.

[245] Steele, Eurídice Martínez, et al. "Ultra-processed foods and added sugars in the US diet: evidence from a nationally representative cross-sectional study." *BMJ open* 6.3 (2016): e009892.

[246] Jenkins, D. J., et al. "Glycemic index of foods: a physiological basis for carbohydrate exchange." *The American journal of clinical nutrition* 34.3 (1981): 362-366.

[247] N Gearhardt, Ashley, et al. "The addiction potential of hyperpalatable foods." *Current drug abuse reviews* 4.3 (2011): 140-145.

[248] Heller, R. F., and Rachael F. Heller. "Hyperinsulinemic obesity and carbohydrate addiction: the missing link is the carbohydrate frequency factor." *Medical hypotheses* 42.5 (1994): 307-312.

[249] Rajaram, Sujatha, and Joan Sabaté. "Nuts, body weight and insulin resistance." *British Journal of Nutrition* 96.S2 (2006): S79-S86.

[250] Bes-Rastrollo, Maira, et al. "Nut consumption and weight gain in a Mediterranean cohort: The SUN study." *Obesity* 15.1 (2007): 107-107.

[251] Claesson, Anna-Lena, et al. "Two weeks of overfeeding with candy, but not peanuts, increases insulin levels and body weight." *Scandinavian journal of clinical and laboratory investigation* 69.5 (2009): 598-605.

[252] Hall, A. P., et al. "Nutrients in Nuts, The Nutritive Value of Fresh and Roasted California Grown Nonpareil Almonds." *Journal of Agricultural and Food Chemistry* 6.5 (1958): 377-382.

[253] Pennington, Jean AT, and Rachel A. Fisher. "Classification of fruits and vegetables." *Journal of Food Composition and Analysis* 22 (2009): S23-S31.

[254] "Oldways Supporters." *Oldways*, Oldways, oldwayspt.org/about-us/funding-support/oldways-supporters.

[255] Jacobs Jr, David R., et al. "Fiber from whole grains, but not refined grains, is inversely associated with all-cause mortality in older women: the Iowa women's health study." *Journal of the American College of Nutrition* 19.sup3 (2000): 326S-330S.

[256] Harris Jackson, Kristina, et al. "Effects of whole and refined grains in a weight-loss diet on markers of metabolic syndrome in individuals with increased waist circumference: a randomized controlled-feeding trial." *The American journal of clinical nutrition* 100.2 (2014): 577-586.

[257] Bertoia, Monica L., et al. "Changes in intake of fruits and vegetables and weight change in United States men and women followed for up to 24 years: analysis from three prospective cohort studies." *PLoS medicine* 12.9 (2015): e1001878.

[258] Faria, Silvia Leite, et al. "Relation between carbohydrate intake and weight loss after bariatric surgery." *Obesity surgery* 19.6 (2009): 708-716.

[259] Fraser, Gary E. "Associations between diet and cancer, ischemic heart disease, and all-cause mortality in non-Hispanic white California Seventh-day Adventists." *The American journal of clinical nutrition* 70.3 (1999): 532s-538s.

[260] Ornish, Dean, et al. "Can lifestyle changes reverse coronary heart disease?: The Lifestyle Heart Trial." *The Lancet* 336.8708 (1990): 129-133.

[261] Pounis, G. D., et al. "Long-term animal-protein consumption is associated with an increased prevalence of diabetes among the elderly: the Mediterranean Islands (MEDIS) study." *Diabetes & metabolism* 36.6 (2010): 484-490.

[262] Lagiou, Pagona, et al. "Low carbohydrate-high protein diet and incidence of cardiovascular diseases in Swedish women: prospective cohort study." *Bmj* 344 (2012):

e4026.

[263] Alkerwi, Ala'A., et al. "The potential impact of animal protein intake on global and abdominal obesity: evidence from the Observation of Cardiovascular Risk Factors in Luxembourg (ORISCAV-LUX) study." *Public health nutrition* 18.10 (2015): 1831-1838.

[264] Bujnowski, Deborah, et al. "Longitudinal association between animal and vegetable protein intake and obesity among men in the United States: the Chicago Western Electric Study." *Journal of the American Dietetic Association* 111.8 (2011): 1150-1155.

[265] Murphy, Karen, et al. "A comparison of regular consumption of fresh lean pork, beef and chicken on body composition: a randomized cross-over trial." *Nutrients* 6.2 (2014): 682-696.

[266] Kamihiro, Sota, et al. "Meat quality and health implications of organic and conventional beef production." *Meat Science* 100 (2015): 306-318.

[267] Bittman, Mark. *Vb6*. Clarkson Potter/Publishers, 2013.

[268] Hill, Graham. "Why I'm a Weekday Vegetarian." *TED*, www.ted.com/talks/graham_hill_weekday_vegetarian?language=en.

[269] Papanikolaou, Yanni, and Victor L. Fulgoni III. "Bean consumption is associated with greater nutrient intake, reduced systolic blood pressure, lower body weight, and a smaller waist circumference in adults: results from the National Health and Nutrition Examination Survey 1999-2002." *Journal of the American College of Nutrition* 27.5 (2008): 569-576.

[270] Simpson, H. C. R., et al. "A high carbohydrate leguminous fibre diet improves all aspects of diabetic control." *The Lancet* 317.8210 (1981): 1-5.

[271] Martinez-Gonzalez, M. A., et al. "Yogurt consumption, weight change and risk of overweight/obesity: the SUN cohort study." *Nutrition, Metabolism and Cardiovascular Diseases* 24.11 (2014): 1189-1196.

[272] Snijder, Marieke B., et al. "Is higher dairy consumption associated with lower body weight and fewer metabolic disturbances? The Hoorn Study." *The American journal of clinical nutrition* 85.4 (2007): 989-995.

[273] Anderson, James W., et al. "Long-term weight maintenance after an intensive weight-loss program." *Journal of the American College of Nutrition* 18.6 (1999): 620-627.

[274] Lewis, Mark C., et al. "Change in liver size and fat content after treatment with Optifast® very low calorie diet." *Obesity surgery* 16.6 (2006): 697-701.

[275] Cassidy, Aedin, Sheila Bingham, and K. D. Setchell. "Biological effects of a diet of soy protein rich in isoflavones on the menstrual cycle of premenopausal women." *The American journal of clinical nutrition* 60.3 (1994): 333-340.

[276] Van Nieuwenhove, Yves, et al. "Preoperative very low-calorie diet and operative outcome after laparoscopic gastric bypass: a randomized multicenter study." *Archives of Surgery* 146.11 (2011): 1300-1305.

[277] Puhl, Rebecca, and Kelly D. Brownell. "Bias, discrimination, and obesity." *Obesity*

research 9.12 (2001): 788-805.

[278] Karlsson, J., et al. "Ten-year trends in health-related quality of life after surgical and conventional treatment for severe obesity: the SOS intervention study." *International journal of obesity* 31.8 (2007): 1248.

[279] Vincent, Heather K., et al. "Rapid changes in gait, musculoskeletal pain, and quality of life after bariatric surgery." *Surgery for Obesity and Related Diseases* 8.3 (2012): 346-354.

[280] Schauer, Philip R., et al. "Bariatric surgery versus intensive medical therapy in obese patients with diabetes." *New England Journal of Medicine* 366.17 (2012): 1567-1576.

[281] Monk, John S., Nancy Dia Nagib, and Wolfgang Stehr. "Pharmaceutical savings after gastric bypass surgery." *Obesity surgery* 14.1 (2004): 13-15.

[282] Flegal, Katherine M., et al. "Association of all-cause mortality with overweight and obesity using standard body mass index categories: a systematic review and meta-analysis." *Jama*309.1 (2013): 71-82.

[283] Christou, Nicolas V., et al. "Surgery decreases long-term mortality, morbidity, and health care use in morbidly obese patients." *Annals of surgery* 240.3 (2004): 416.

Made in the USA
Columbia, SC
10 October 2021